LOW CARB HIGH PROTEIN COOKBOOK FOR BEGINNERS

Delicious Low-Carb, High-Protein Meals to Lose Weight and Build Muscle with Ease in Just 28 Days I 60-Day Meal Plan to Stay on Track Included

EMMA STONE

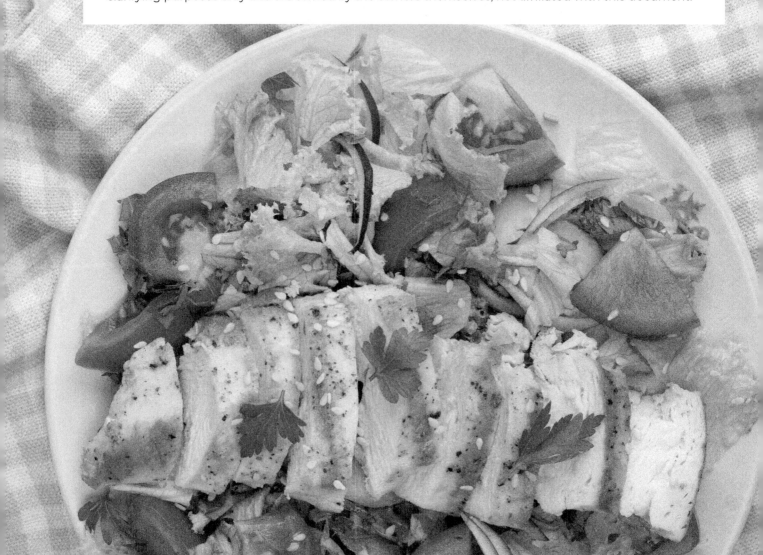

Table of Contents

CHAPTER 5
SNACKS AND SMOOTHIES TO KEEP YOU ON TRACK

CLAIM YOUR EXCLUSIVE BONUSES!

Enhance Your Low-Carb Journey with These Essential Tools – Free for You!

1. **Quick Low-Carb Snack Guide** – Fast, delicious, and easy-to-make snacks that will keep you satisfied and on track.
2. **Weekly Meal Planning Template** – Simplify your week with a clear plan for every meal, so you never have to wonder what to eat next.
3. **Family-Friendly Recipe Collection** – Enjoy healthy, low-carb meals that your whole family will love without having to prepare separate dishes.

Don't Miss Out – Take Full Advantage of These FREE Resources to Simplify Your Life and Supercharge Your Results!

Scroll to the End of the Book and Scan the QR CODE to Instantly download Your EXCLUSIVE BONUS

Introduction

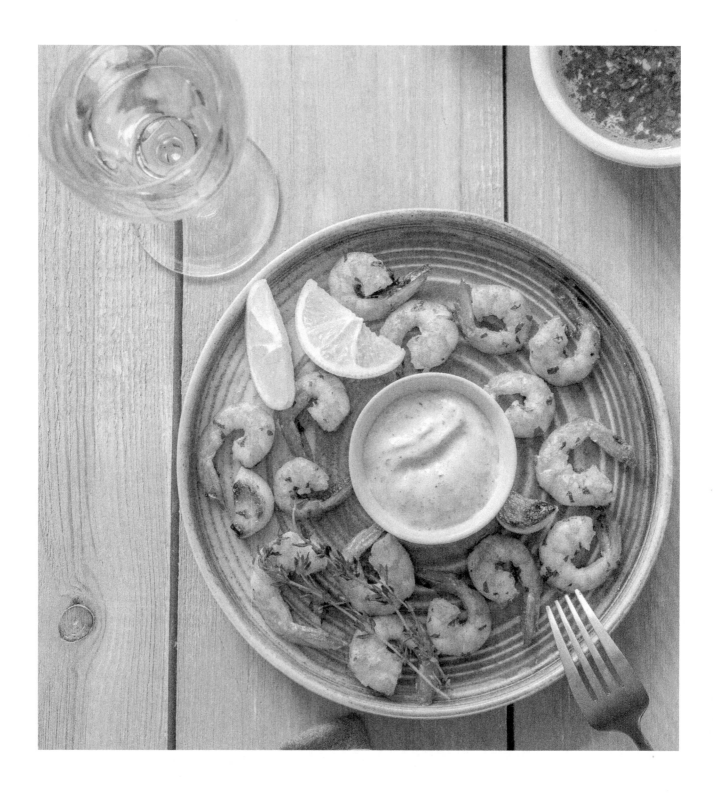

In today's fast-paced world, finding a diet that fits seamlessly into a busy life while delivering real, lasting results can feel like a challenge. You've likely tried different approaches to eating—some restrictive, others complicated—and been left feeling frustrated or drained. This book is designed to change that, offering a simple yet powerful way to lose weight, gain muscle, and boost your energy, all without spending hours in the kitchen or sacrificing taste.

Many of us, perhaps even you, have tried various diets in the past. Whether it was keto, paleo, or a low-fat diet, the promises of quick results were enticing, but the reality often felt far more demanding. Maybe you found yourself feeling deprived of foods you love, or maybe the meal prep took so long that you started to resent spending time in the kitchen. It's frustrating to commit to something, only to see that it doesn't fit with your lifestyle. That's why this book takes a different approach, making sure that the recipes and strategies offered can realistically fit into your everyday routine.

This isn't just another diet book. It's not about quick fixes, impossible meal plans, or cooking gourmet meals every night. This is a guide for real people with real lives—people who are juggling work, family, personal commitments, and, sometimes, simply the struggle to keep their heads above water. If that sounds like you, then you're in the right place. The Low Carb High Protein Cookbook for Beginners is designed to offer you a sustainable and delicious way to achieve your health goals without adding extra stress to your life.

What is the Low Carb High Protein Diet and Why It Works

The Low Carb High Protein diet focuses on reducing the intake of carbohydrates while increasing the consumption of protein-rich foods. But unlike many other diets that suggest drastically cutting out entire food groups, this one is far more balanced and realistic. It doesn't demand that you give up all your favorite foods, nor does it require that you meticulously count calories or carbs every day. Instead, it's based on understanding how the body uses macronutrients and learning to make smarter food choices that will keep you full, energized, and satisfied.

To understand why this diet works, it's helpful to look at how your body processes different types of foods. Carbohydrates, especially refined carbs like white bread, pasta, and sugar, are quickly broken down into glucose in the body. This glucose gives you an immediate spike in energy, but as anyone who's ever experienced a sugar crash can tell you, that energy doesn't last. After the initial surge, blood sugar levels drop rapidly, leaving you feeling tired, sluggish, and hungry again. This often leads to cravings for more carbs, creating a cycle of energy spikes and crashes that can be tough to break.

When you reduce your intake of carbs, particularly the refined ones, and replace them with protein and healthy fats, you stabilize your blood sugar levels. Instead of riding the roller coaster of energy highs and lows, your body begins to burn fat for fuel, which leads to more sustained energy throughout the day. You won't find yourself starving between meals or experiencing that mid-afternoon slump where you feel like you need another cup of coffee just to keep going.

Protein, on the other hand, is the body's building block. It's essential not only for muscle repair and growth but also for keeping you feeling full and satisfied. Protein has a higher thermic effect than fats or carbs, meaning your body uses more energy to digest it, which in turn helps you burn more calories. High-protein foods also help preserve lean muscle mass as you lose weight, ensuring that the pounds you shed come from fat, not muscle.

A Low Carb High Protein diet is also incredibly flexible. You don't need to cut out whole food groups or give up on the meals you love. Instead, it's about making smarter choices—choosing lean proteins like chicken, fish, and plant-based options, and pairing them with non-starchy vegetables and healthy fats like avocado and olive oil. It's a way of eating that can easily fit into your life, whether you're cooking for yourself, your family, or dealing with unpredictable work schedules.

This diet isn't about deprivation or complicated rules. It's about finding balance. When you focus on eating foods that nourish your body and provide sustained energy, you'll naturally feel more satisfied and less likely to reach for unhealthy snacks or comfort foods.

Why This Book is Different

What sets this book apart from other diet books is its emphasis on flexibility and sustainability. Many diet plans start with good intentions, but they quickly become unsustainable when they demand too much time, too much effort, or too much sacrifice. That's why so many people find themselves giving up after a few weeks, reverting back to old habits, and feeling like they've failed. But the truth is, it's not the person who's failing—it's the plan that wasn't realistic to begin with.

This book takes a different approach. It's not about following a rigid meal plan that dictates every bite you take for the next two months. Instead, it offers you a flexible structure that you can adapt to your own needs and preferences. The recipes in this book are designed to be quick and easy, with most of them taking under 30 minutes to prepare. That means you won't spend hours in the kitchen, and you won't feel overwhelmed by complex recipes that require dozens of ingredients you don't have on hand.

Another key feature of this book is the customizable 60-day meal plan. Unlike traditional meal plans that offer little room for personalization, this one is designed to work with your life, not against it. You can swap out ingredients you don't like, adjust portion sizes based on your goals, and even make modifications for your family members, ensuring that everyone at the table can enjoy the same meal. If you have a particularly busy week, you can choose the quickest recipes, or if you have more time, you can prepare meals in advance.

The book also includes over 100 recipes that focus on taste, nutrition, and ease of preparation. Whether you're new to cooking or an experienced home chef, you'll find recipes that are simple yet flavorful, and above all, practical. And because this book is all about flexibility, you won't be stuck following a rigid plan. Instead, you'll have the freedom to choose the meals that work best for you and your family. You'll also find downloadable resources like snack guides and meal planning templates that make it even easier to stay on track.

This is not just another fad diet book that leaves you feeling frustrated and hungry. This is a guide designed for real life—your life—and it gives you the tools you need to make healthy eating a habit, not a chore. The focus is on sustainability, which means you'll be able to stick with these changes long enough to see real, lasting results.

Who is This Book For

This book is for anyone who's ever struggled to balance healthy eating with a busy life. If you're someone who juggles work, family, and personal commitments, and you often feel like there aren't enough hours in the day to take care of yourself, then this book is for you. You don't need to be a health expert or a fitness guru to benefit from the strategies in this book. All you need is a willingness to make small, manageable changes that fit into your current lifestyle.

If you've tried diets in the past and found them too restrictive or complicated, this book offers a fresh approach. It's designed for beginners and anyone looking for a straightforward, no-nonsense guide to better eating. You won't find rigid rules or unrealistic expectations here. Instead, you'll find recipes and tips that are easy to follow and won't take hours of your time. And because this book is rooted in flexibility, you'll be able to adapt it to your needs, ensuring that you can stick with it even when life gets hectic.

The recipes in this book are also family-friendly, meaning you won't have to cook separate meals for yourself and your family. Whether you're cooking for picky eaters or trying to please a crowd, you'll find options that everyone can enjoy. The focus is on creating meals that are healthy, satisfying, and delicious, so you won't feel like you're sacrificing flavor for the sake of your diet.

In the end, this book is for anyone who wants to feel more in control of their health and nutrition. Whether your goal is to lose weight, build muscle, or simply feel more energized throughout the day, the Low Carb High Protein Cookbook for Beginners is here to guide you. This is your opportunity to finally achieve the results you've been striving for, without the frustration and without the stress.

CHAPTER 1

The Basics of Low Carb and High Protein

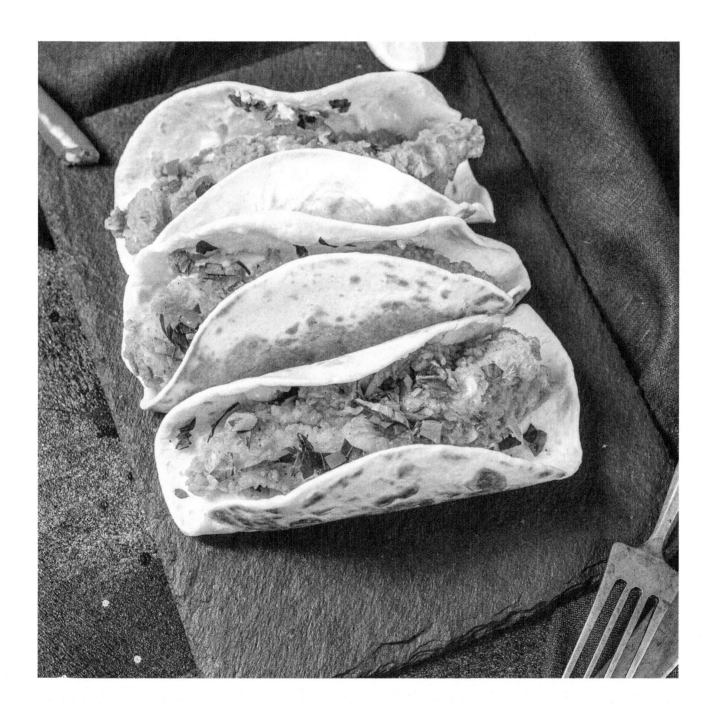

When it comes to adopting a healthier lifestyle, understanding the basics is crucial. The Low Carb High Protein diet is not just a trend but a well-rounded approach that can make a significant difference in how you feel, look, and perform daily. In this chapter, we'll dive into the essential concepts of this diet, helping you grasp what makes it effective and, more importantly, sustainable.

Understanding Macronutrients: Carbs, Protein, and Fat

To fully embrace the Low Carb High Protein diet, it's essential to understand the building blocks of nutrition—macronutrients. These are carbohydrates, proteins, and fats, and each plays a unique role in fueling your body.

Carbohydrates are often viewed as the body's primary energy source. When you consume carbs, they break down into glucose, which provides quick energy. However, in our modern diets, we often consume too many refined carbs, which can lead to rapid spikes and crashes in blood sugar. These fluctuations leave us craving more sugar and carbs, starting a cycle that's hard to break. This is why reducing carbs, particularly the processed kinds, can help stabilize energy levels.

Protein, on the other hand, is like the body's repair crew. It builds and maintains muscles, helps with recovery after physical activity, and provides a longer-lasting feeling of fullness. When you increase protein intake, you not only support muscle growth but also boost your metabolism. This is because digesting protein requires more energy compared to carbs and fat, which means you burn more calories simply by eating it.

Then there are fats, which for years were misunderstood and avoided in many diets. However, healthy fats—like those found in avocados, olive oil, and fatty fish—are essential for brain function, hormone production, and maintaining a healthy heart. In a low-carb, high-protein diet, fats help provide steady energy without the blood sugar spikes and crashes that come from carbs.

By understanding the roles of these macronutrients, you can start to make smarter food choices that support your health goals. When you focus on the right balance of protein, healthy fats, and limited carbs, your body works more efficiently, burning fat for fuel and keeping you energized.

The Benefits of the Low Carb, High Protein Diet

Now that we've covered what carbs, proteins, and fats do in your body, let's talk about why the Low Carb High Protein diet is so effective and beneficial. At its core, this diet offers a balanced way to achieve weight loss, maintain muscle, and improve overall health.

One of the biggest benefits is its impact on **weight loss**. By lowering carb intake and increasing protein, your body is prompted to use fat stores for energy. This process, known as ketosis, is why low-carb diets are often so successful for fat loss, particularly around the abdomen. Unlike many diets that result in both fat and muscle loss, high-protein intake ensures that while you're shedding fat, your muscle mass stays intact. This is crucial because muscle helps burn more calories, even when you're at rest.

Another key advantage is the **stabilization of blood sugar levels**. With fewer refined carbs, your body avoids the dramatic spikes and dips in blood sugar that can lead to energy crashes and cravings. This makes it easier to avoid snacking on unhealthy foods and keeps you feeling more balanced throughout the day.

The diet also supports **muscle building and maintenance**. Protein is essential for muscle repair and growth, which is why this diet is particularly beneficial for those who are physically active or looking to tone their body. Even if you're not aiming for a bodybuilder physique, maintaining lean muscle is crucial for a healthy metabolism and long-term weight management.

A lesser-known benefit is the **boost in sustained energy**. Because your body isn't relying on sugar for quick energy, it turns to fats and protein, which provide a more consistent energy source. This means no more afternoon slumps or post-meal crashes. You'll feel steady, alert, and energized throughout the day, which is a major win for anyone balancing work, family, and personal life.

Finally, by reducing the intake of processed carbs and sugars, the Low Carb High Protein diet can also contribute to **improved heart health**. Eating more whole, unprocessed foods—rich in healthy fats and protein—helps lower bad cholesterol, reduce inflammation, and stabilize blood pressure, which are all important factors for long-term cardiovascular health.

How to Structure a Low Carb, High Protein Meal

With a good understanding of how this diet works, the next step is learning how to structure your meals. It's simpler than you might think, and once you get into the rhythm of it, meal planning becomes second nature.

The first rule is to always **start with protein**. Whether it's a lean chicken breast, a piece of fish, or plant-based options like tofu or lentils, protein should be the anchor of every meal. This will help keep you full and provide the building blocks your body needs for muscle maintenance and energy.

Next, add **non-starchy vegetables**. Think leafy greens, broccoli, zucchini, bell peppers, or cauliflower. These vegetables are nutrient-dense, low in carbs, and high in fiber, which helps with digestion and keeps you feeling full. They also provide essential vitamins and minerals that support your overall health.

Incorporating **healthy fats** is key to making your meal satisfying. Avocados, nuts, seeds, and olive oil are all excellent choices. Fats not only add flavor but also help your body absorb the fat-soluble vitamins in your meal.

Lastly, while this diet limits carbs, you can still enjoy **moderate portions of complex carbohydrates**. Instead of reaching for bread or pasta, opt for nutri-ent-dense carbs like sweet potatoes, quinoa, or legumes, but keep portions small. These will give you the fiber and slow-burning energy you need without spiking your blood sugar.

Common Mistakes and How to Avoid Them

Even with the best intentions, it's easy to make mistakes when starting a new diet. One of the most common mistakes people make on the Low Carb High Protein diet is **not eating enough protein**. It can be tempting to skimp on protein, especially if you're in a hurry or don't feel like cooking, but getting enough protein is essential for keeping your metabolism running efficiently and your muscles strong. Aim to include a serving of protein in every meal.

Another common pitfall is **hidden carbs**. Many processed foods, including sauces, dressings, and snacks, contain added sugars or starches that can add up quickly. It's important to check food labels and, when possible, prepare your meals at home using whole ingredients. This will help you avoid unnecessary carbs that could hinder your progress.

Many people also still have a lingering fear of **healthy fats**. Years of misinformation have led us to believe that eating fat makes you fat, but this simply isn't true when you're eating the right kinds of fats. Avocados, nuts, olive oil, and fatty fish are all excellent choices that support heart health and keep you satisfied.

Lastly, it's important to stay **hydrated**. A low-carb diet can sometimes cause the body to lose more water, especially in the early stages, which can lead to dehydration if you're not careful. Drinking plenty of water not only helps keep you hydrated but also supports digestion and helps you feel more full throughout the day.

Tracking Your Progress

Tracking your progress is one of the most important steps in ensuring long-term success on any diet. This isn't just about watching the numbers on the scale, though that can be helpful. It's about recognizing the changes in how you feel, how your clothes fit, and your energy levels.

One simple way to track progress is by **measuring your food intake**, especially in the beginning. This helps you understand portion sizes and ensures you're getting enough protein and staying within your carb limits. Over time, you'll become more intuitive about portion sizes and won't need to measure as often.

Another great way to track your progress is by **monitoring your weight and body measurements**. The scale isn't always the best indicator of success, especially if you're building muscle while losing fat, so it's important to take measurements of your waist, hips, and other key areas to see where your body is changing.

Paying attention to how you feel on a daily basis is also crucial. **Energy levels, mood, and sleep quality** can all be indicators of how well the diet is working for you. You might notice that you're feeling more alert, less bloated, or more energized throughout the day—these are all signs that your body is adjusting positively.

Lastly, as you track your progress, be open to making adjustments. If you notice that your energy levels are dipping, you might need to slightly increase your carb intake. If you feel like you're losing muscle mass, add more protein. The goal is to find a balance that works best for your unique body and lifestyle.

With this foundation, you're ready to move forward confidently with the Low Carb High Protein diet. By understanding macronutrients, structuring your meals effectively, avoiding common mistakes, and tracking your progress, you'll be able to create lasting change that supports your health goals. This diet isn't just about quick fixes—it's a long-term approach to feeling stronger, healthier, and more in control of your well-being.

CHAPTER 2
Breakfast Recipes to Kickstart Your Day

Breakfast is the most important meal of the day, and with the right ingredients, it can set you up for success. In this chapter, we're focusing on high-protein, low-carb breakfasts that are not only delicious but also quick and easy to prepare. These recipes are perfect for busy mornings, ensuring that you start your day fueled, energized, and satisfied.

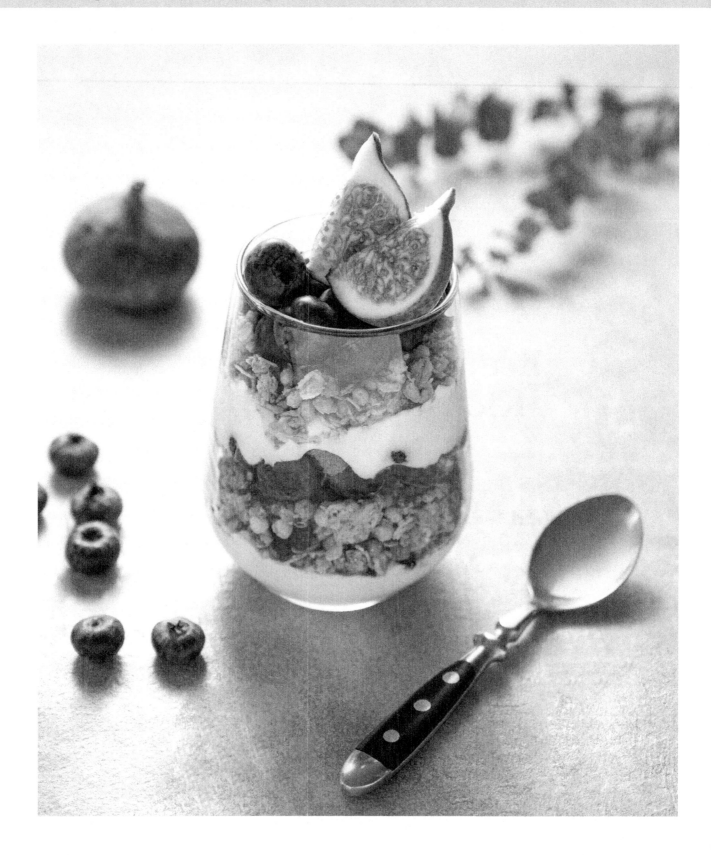

1. Classic Protein Omelette

Prep Time: 5 minutes   **Cook Time: 5 minutes**   **Serves: 1**

INGREDIENTS:

- 2 large eggs
- 1/4 cup shredded cheese (cheddar or your choice)
- 1/4 cup spinach, chopped
- Salt and pepper to taste
- 1 tsp olive oil

INSTRUCTIONS:

1. Beat the eggs in a bowl and season with salt and pepper.
2. Heat olive oil in a skillet over medium heat.
3. Pour in the eggs and let them cook for 2-3 minutes until the edges set.
4. Sprinkle cheese and spinach on one half of the omelette and fold the other half over.
5. Cook for another minute until the cheese melts. Serve hot.

Nutritional Facts (Per Serving):

Calories: 260 Protein: 17g Carbohydrates: 2g Fat: 21g

2. Low-Carb Breakfast Casserole

Prep Time: 10 minutes   **Cook Time: 25 minutes**   **Serves: 4**

INGREDIENTS:

- 8 large eggs
- 1/2 lb ground turkey or sausage
- 1/2 cup shredded cheese (cheddar or mozzarella)
- 1/2 cup bell peppers, diced
- 1/4 cup onion, diced
- Salt and pepper to taste

INSTRUCTIONS:

1. Preheat your oven to 375°F (190°C).
2. In a skillet, cook ground turkey or sausage until browned.
3. In a large bowl, whisk the eggs and mix in cheese, bell peppers, onion, and cooked turkey or sausage.
4. Pour the mixture into a greased baking dish and bake for 20-25 minutes until fully cooked.
5. Let cool slightly before serving.

Nutritional Facts (Per Serving):

Calories: 300 Protein: 22g Carbohydrates: 3g Fat: 22g

3. Avocado and Egg Bowl

Prep Time: 5 minutes   **Cook Time: 10 minutes**   **Serves: 1**

INGREDIENTS:

- 1 ripe avocado
- 2 eggs
- Salt and pepper to taste
- 1 tbsp olive oil

INSTRUCTIONS:

1. Slice the avocado in half and remove the pit.
2. Heat olive oil in a pan and fry the eggs to your liking.
3. Place the fried eggs into the avocado halves and season with salt and pepper. Serve immediately.

Nutritional Facts (Per Serving):

Calories: 400 Protein: 12g Carbohydrates: 9g Fat: 36g

4. Egg Muffins with Veggies

Prep Time: 10 minutes   **Cook Time: 20 minutes**   **Serves: 6**

INGREDIENTS:

- 6 large eggs
- 1/2 cup spinach, chopped
- 1/2 cup bell peppers, diced
- 1/4 cup shredded cheese (optional)
- Salt and pepper to taste

INSTRUCTIONS:

1. Preheat your oven to 350°F (175°C).
2. In a bowl, whisk eggs and season with salt and pepper.
3. Mix in spinach, bell peppers, and cheese.
4. Pour the mixture into a greased muffin tin.
5. Bake for 18-20 minutes until set. Serve warm or store for later.

Nutritional Facts (Per Serving):

Calories: 120 Protein: 10g Carbohydrates: 2g Fat: 9g

5. Greek Yogurt Protein Parfait

Prep Time: 5 minutes   **Cook Time: None**   **Serves: 1**

INGREDIENTS:

- 1/2 cup plain Greek yogurt
- 1/4 cup mixed berries (blueberries, raspberries, etc.)
- 1 tbsp chia seeds
- 1 tbsp unsweetened coconut flakes

INSTRUCTIONS:

1. Layer Greek yogurt, berries, chia seeds, and coconut flakes in a bowl or glass.
2. Serve immediately or store in the refrigerator for a chilled treat.

Nutritional Facts (Per Serving):

Calories: 180 Protein: 15g Carbohydrates: 10g Fat: 7g

6. Almond Flour Pancakes

Prep Time: 5 minutes   **Cook Time: 10 minutes**   **Serves: 2**

INGREDIENTS:

- 1/2 cup almond flour
- 2 large eggs
- 1 tbsp coconut oil
- 1/2 tsp baking powder
- 1/4 tsp vanilla extract

INSTRUCTIONS:

1. In a bowl, whisk together all ingredients until smooth.
2. Heat a skillet over medium heat and grease with coconut oil.
3. Pour batter onto the skillet, forming small pancakes.
4. Cook for 2-3 minutes on each side until golden brown. Serve with a low-carb syrup or fresh berries.

Nutritional Facts (Per Serving):

Calories: 250 Protein: 12g Carbohydrates: 6g Fat: 21g

7. Keto-Friendly Waffles

Prep Time: 10 minutes   **Cook Time: 10 minutes**   **Serves: 2**

INGREDIENTS:

- 1/2 cup almond flour
- 2 large eggs
- 1 tbsp melted butter
- 1/2 tsp baking powder
- 1/4 tsp cinnamon

INSTRUCTIONS:

1. Preheat a waffle iron.
2. In a bowl, mix together all ingredients until smooth.
3. Pour the batter into the waffle iron and cook until golden brown. Serve with sugar-free syrup or fresh berries.

Nutritional Facts (Per Serving):

Calories: 280 Protein: 10g Carbohydrates: 5g Fat: 24g

8. Spinach and Feta Frittata

Prep Time: 10 minutes   **Cook Time: 15 minutes**   **Serves: 4**

INGREDIENTS:

- 6 large eggs
- 1 cup spinach, chopped
- 1/4 cup crumbled feta cheese
- Salt and pepper to taste

INSTRUCTIONS:

1. Preheat your oven to 375°F (190°C).
2. In a bowl, whisk eggs and season with salt and pepper.
3. Stir in spinach and feta.
4. Pour the mixture into a greased oven-safe skillet and bake for 12-15 minutes until set. Serve hot.

Nutritional Facts (Per Serving):

Calories: 220 Protein: 14g Carbohydrates: 2g Fat: 17g

9. Smoked Salmon & Cream Cheese Roll

Prep Time: 5 minutes   **Cook Time: None**   **Serves: 1**

INGREDIENTS:

- 3 slices smoked salmon
- 2 tbsp cream cheese
- 1 tbsp chopped chives

INSTRUCTIONS:

1. Spread cream cheese onto each slice of smoked salmon.
2. Sprinkle with chopped chives and roll up tightly.
3. Serve as is or chilled for a refreshing breakfast option.

Nutritional Facts (Per Serving):

Calories: 200 Protein: 12g Carbohydrates: 2g Fat: 16g

10. Low-Carb Breakfast Burrito

Prep Time: 5 minutes   **Cook Time: 5 minutes**   **Serves: 1**

INGREDIENTS:

- 2 large eggs
- 1/4 cup shredded cheese
- 1/4 avocado, sliced
- 1 low-carb tortilla
- Salt and pepper to taste

INSTRUCTIONS:

1. Scramble the eggs in a skillet until fully cooked.
2. Lay the scrambled eggs, cheese, and avocado in the center of the tortilla.
3. Roll up the tortilla and serve immediately.

Nutritional Facts (Per Serving):

Calories: 300 Protein: 18g Carbohydrates: 7g Fat: 22g

11. Chia Seed Pudding with Berries

Prep Time: 5 minutes   **Cook Time: None**   **Serves: 2**

INGREDIENTS:

- 1/4 cup chia seeds
- 1 cup unsweetened almond milk
- 1/4 cup mixed berries
- 1 tsp vanilla extract

INSTRUCTIONS:

1. Mix chia seeds, almond milk, and vanilla extract in a bowl.
2. Let the mixture sit for at least 2 hours or overnight to thicken.
3. Top with fresh berries and serve.

Nutritional Facts (Per Serving):

Calories: 180 Protein: 6g Carbohydrates: 10g Fat: 12g

12. Turkey and Cheese Breakfast Wrap

Prep Time: 5 minutes   **Cook Time: 5 minutes**   **Serves: 1**

INGREDIENTS:

- 2 slices turkey breast
- 1 slice cheese (cheddar or your choice)
- 1 tbsp mustard or mayonnaise
- 1 low-carb tortilla

INSTRUCTIONS:

1. Layer turkey, cheese, and mustard or mayo on the tortilla.
2. Roll up tightly and serve cold or warm.

Nutritional Facts (Per Serving):

Calories: 250 Protein: 18g Carbohydrates: 6g Fat: 16g

13. Low-Carb Granola with Nuts and Seeds

Prep Time: 5 minutes   Cook Time: 10 minutes   Serves: 4

INGREDIENTS:

- 1/2 cup almonds, chopped
- 1/2 cup sunflower seeds
- 1/4 cup unsweetened coconut flakes
- 1 tbsp coconut oil
- 1 tsp cinnamon

INSTRUCTIONS:

1. Preheat your oven to 325°F (160°C).
2. Mix all ingredients together in a bowl.
3. Spread the mixture on a baking sheet and bake for 10-12 minutes until golden. Let cool before serving.

Nutritional Facts (Per Serving):

Calories: 200 Protein: 6g Carbohydrates: 5g Fat: 18g

14. Zucchini Fritters with Egg

Prep Time: 10 minutes   Cook Time: 15 minutes   Serves: 2

INGREDIENTS:

- 1 medium zucchini, grated
- 1 egg
- 1/4 cup almond flour
- 1 tbsp olive oil

INSTRUCTIONS:

1. Squeeze the excess moisture out of the grated zucchini.
2. In a bowl, mix zucchini, egg, and almond flour.
3. Heat olive oil in a pan and spoon the mixture to form fritters. Cook for 3-4 minutes on each side. Serve hot.

Nutritional Facts (Per Serving):

Calories: 180 Protein: 6g Carbohydrates: 4g Fat: 14g

15. Cottage Cheese and Berry Bowl

Prep Time: 5 minutes　　　　　**Cook Time: None**　　　　　**Serves: 1**

INGREDIENTS:

- 1/2 cup cottage cheese
- 1/4 cup mixed berries
- 1 tbsp chia seeds

INSTRUCTIONS:

1. Combine cottage cheese and berries in a bowl.
2. Sprinkle chia seeds on top and serve.

Nutritional Facts (Per Serving):

Calories: 150 Protein: 10g Carbohydrates: 8g Fat: 7g

CHAPTER 3

Lunch Recipes to Keep You Satisfied

Lunchtime is when you need a satisfying meal to fuel you through the rest of your day. These low-carb, high-protein lunch recipes will help you stay full and energized without the sluggishness that often comes after a heavy, carb-loaded meal. From salads and wraps to protein-packed bowls, these recipes are easy to prepare and perfect for a busy lifestyle.

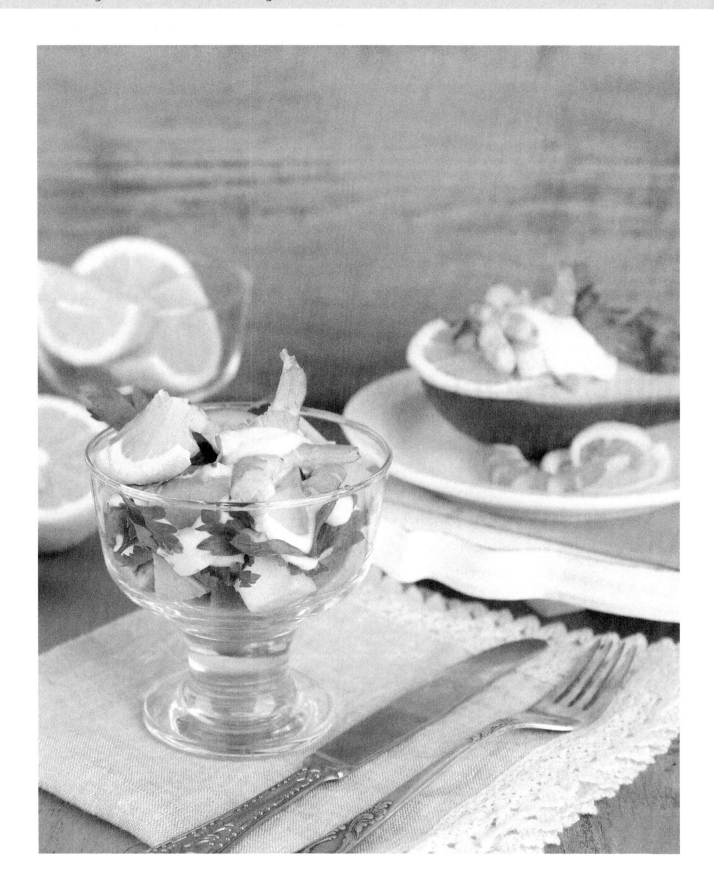

16. Chicken Caesar Salad Wrap

Prep Time: 10 minutes   **Cook Time: None**   **Serves: 1**

INGREDIENTS:

- 1 grilled chicken breast, sliced
- 1 low-carb tortilla
- 1 tbsp Caesar dressing
- 1/4 cup romaine lettuce, chopped
- 1 tbsp grated Parmesan cheese

INSTRUCTIONS:

1. Lay the tortilla flat and spread Caesar dressing evenly.
2. Add chicken slices, lettuce, and Parmesan cheese.
3. Wrap tightly and enjoy.

Nutritional Facts (Per Serving):

Calories: 350 Protein: 30g Carbohydrates: 7g Fat: 22g

17. Grilled Lemon Garlic Chicken Salad

Prep Time: 10 minutes   **Cook Time: 10 minutes**   **Serves: 2**

INGREDIENTS:

- 2 grilled chicken breasts
- 4 cups mixed greens
- 1/2 avocado, sliced
- 1 tbsp olive oil
- 1 tbsp lemon juice
- 1 clove garlic, minced
- Salt and pepper to taste

INSTRUCTIONS:

1. Grill the chicken breasts until cooked through, then slice.
2. In a bowl, toss mixed greens, avocado, olive oil, lemon juice, garlic, salt, and pepper.
3. Top with grilled chicken slices and serve.

Nutritional Facts (Per Serving):

Calories: 420 Protein: 32g Carbohydrates: 6g Fat: 30g

18. Turkey and Avocado Lettuce Wraps

Prep Time: 5 minutes   **Cook Time: None**   **Serves: 1**

INGREDIENTS:

- 4 slices deli turkey
- 1/2 avocado, sliced
- 4 large romaine lettuce leaves
- 1 tbsp mayonnaise

INSTRUCTIONS:

1. Spread mayonnaise on the turkey slices.
2. Lay turkey and avocado slices on each lettuce leaf.
3. Roll up and enjoy.

Nutritional Facts (Per Serving):

Calories: 250 Protein: 16g Carbohydrates: 5g Fat: 19g

19. Shrimp and Avocado Salad

Prep Time: 10 minutes   **Cook Time: 5 minutes**   **Serves: 2**

INGREDIENTS:

- 12 shrimp, peeled and deveined
- 1/2 avocado, diced
- 2 cups mixed greens
- 1 tbsp olive oil
- 1 tbsp lemon juice
- Salt and pepper to taste

INSTRUCTIONS:

1. Heat a skillet over medium heat and sauté shrimp for 3-4 minutes until pink.
2. In a bowl, toss mixed greens, avocado, olive oil, lemon juice, salt, and pepper.
3. Top with shrimp and serve.

Nutritional Facts (Per Serving):

Calories: 300 Protein: 25g Carbohydrates: 5g Fat: 20g

20. Low-Carb Cobb Salad

Prep Time: 10 minutes   **Cook Time: None**   **Serves: 2**

INGREDIENTS:

- 2 hard-boiled eggs, chopped
- 1/2 avocado, diced
- 2 cups mixed greens
- 4 slices cooked bacon, crumbled
- 1/4 cup blue cheese, crumbled
- 1 grilled chicken breast, sliced
- 2 tbsp olive oil
- 1 tbsp red wine vinegar

INSTRUCTIONS:

1. Arrange mixed greens in a bowl and top with eggs, avocado, bacon, blue cheese, and chicken.
2. Drizzle with olive oil and red wine vinegar. Serve immediately.

Nutritional Facts (Per Serving):

Calories: 450 Protein: 30g Carbohydrates: 5g Fat: 35g

21. Greek Chicken Salad with Feta

Prep Time: 10 minutes   **Cook Time: 10 minutes**   **Serves: 2**

INGREDIENTS:

- 1 grilled chicken breast, diced
- 2 cups mixed greens
- 1/4 cup feta cheese, crumbled
- 1/4 cucumber, sliced
- 1/4 cup cherry tomatoes, halved
- 1 tbsp olive oil
- 1 tbsp lemon juice
- Salt and pepper to taste

INSTRUCTIONS:

1. In a large bowl, combine greens, feta, cucumber, and cherry tomatoes.
2. Top with diced chicken, olive oil, lemon juice, salt, and pepper.
3. Toss lightly and serve.

Nutritional Facts (Per Serving):

Calories: 350 Protein: 28g Carbohydrates: 6g Fat: 24g

22. Tuna Salad Lettuce Wraps

Prep Time: 5 minutes   **Cook Time: None**   **Serves: 1**

INGREDIENTS:

- 1 can tuna, drained
- 2 tbsp mayonnaise
- 1/4 cup celery, diced
- 4 large lettuce leaves
- Salt and pepper to taste

INSTRUCTIONS:

1. In a bowl, mix tuna, mayonnaise, celery, salt, and pepper.
2. Spoon the tuna salad onto lettuce leaves and roll them up.
3. Serve immediately.

Nutritional Facts (Per Serving):

Calories: 220 Protein: 24g Carbohydrates: 3g Fat: 12g

23. Turkey and Veggie Roll-ups

Prep Time: 10 minutes   **Cook Time: None**   **Serves: 2**

INGREDIENTS:

- 4 slices turkey breast
- 4 slices cucumber
- 4 slices red bell pepper
- 2 tbsp cream cheese
- 1 tbsp mustard

INSTRUCTIONS:

1. Spread cream cheese and mustard on each turkey slice.
2. Add cucumber and bell pepper slices, then roll up the turkey.
3. Secure with toothpicks if needed and serve.

Nutritional Facts (Per Serving):

Calories: 200 Protein: 18g Carbohydrates: 5g Fat: 14g

24. Mediterranean Chickpea Salad (Low-Carb)

Prep Time: 10 minutes　　　**Cook Time: None**　　　**Serves: 2**

INGREDIENTS:

- 1/2 cup canned chickpeas, rinsed and drained
- 1/4 cup feta cheese, crumbled
- 1/4 cup cucumber, diced
- 1/4 cup cherry tomatoes, halved
- 1 tbsp olive oil
- 1 tbsp lemon juice
- Salt and pepper to taste

INSTRUCTIONS:

1. In a bowl, combine chickpeas, feta, cucumber, and cherry tomatoes.
2. Drizzle with olive oil, lemon juice, salt, and pepper. Toss well.
3. Serve chilled or at room temperature.

Nutritional Facts (Per Serving):

Calories: 250 Protein: 12g Carbohydrates: 20g Fat: 14g

25. Cauliflower Rice with Grilled Chicken

Prep Time: 10 minutes　　　**Cook Time: 10 minutes**　　　**Serves: 2**

INGREDIENTS:

- 1 cup cauliflower rice
- 2 grilled chicken breasts, sliced
- 1 tbsp olive oil
- 1 clove garlic, minced
- Salt and pepper to taste

INSTRUCTIONS:

1. Heat olive oil in a pan and sauté garlic until fragrant.
2. Add cauliflower rice and cook for 5-7 minutes until tender.
3. Serve with grilled chicken slices on top and season with salt and pepper.

Nutritional Facts (Per Serving):

Calories: 320 Protein: 30g Carbohydrates: 6g Fat: 20g

26. Grilled Steak and Veggie Bowl

Prep Time: 10 minutes   **Cook Time: 10 minutes**   **Serves: 2**

INGREDIENTS:

- 2 small steaks, grilled and sliced
- 1/2 cup bell peppers, sliced
- 1/2 cup zucchini, sliced
- 2 tbsp olive oil
- Salt and pepper to taste

INSTRUCTIONS:

1. Heat olive oil in a skillet and sauté bell peppers and zucchini until tender.
2. Place grilled steak slices over the sautéed veggies and serve.

Nutritional Facts (Per Serving):

Calories: 400 Protein: 30g Carbohydrates: 8g Fat: 30g

27. Low-Carb Chicken Fajita Bowl

Prep Time: 10 minutes   **Cook Time: 10 minutes**   **Serves: 2**

INGREDIENTS:

- 2 grilled chicken breasts, sliced
- 1/2 bell pepper, sliced
- 1/2 onion, sliced
- 1 tbsp olive oil
- 1 tsp cumin
- 1 tsp chili powder
- Salt and pepper to taste

INSTRUCTIONS:

1. Heat olive oil in a pan and sauté bell pepper and onion until tender.
2. Add sliced chicken, cumin, chili powder, salt, and pepper. Cook for 2-3 minutes.
3. Serve in bowls with optional toppings like sour cream or guacamole.

Nutritional Facts (Per Serving):

Calories: 350 Protein: 32g Carbohydrates: 6g Fat: 22g

28. Sesame Ginger Chicken Salad

Prep Time: 10 minutes   **Cook Time: 10 minutes**   **Serves: 2**

INGREDIENTS:

- 2 grilled chicken breasts, sliced
- 2 cups mixed greens
- 1 tbsp sesame oil
- 1 tbsp soy sauce (or tamari)
- 1 tsp grated ginger
- 1 tbsp rice vinegar
- 1 tbsp sesame seeds

INSTRUCTIONS:

1. In a small bowl, whisk sesame oil, soy sauce, ginger, and rice vinegar.
2. Toss mixed greens with the dressing and top with sliced chicken and sesame seeds.
3. Serve immediately.

Nutritional Facts (Per Serving):

Calories: 340 Protein: 30g Carbohydrates: 4g Fat: 22g

29. Caprese Salad with Chicken

Prep Time: 5 minutes   **Cook Time: None**   **Serves: 2**

INGREDIENTS:

- 1 grilled chicken breast, sliced
- 1/4 cup mozzarella balls
- 1/2 cup cherry tomatoes, halved
- 1 tbsp balsamic vinegar
- 1 tbsp olive oil
- Fresh basil leaves

INSTRUCTIONS:

1. Arrange chicken slices, mozzarella balls, and cherry tomatoes on a plate.
2. Drizzle with balsamic vinegar and olive oil.
3. Garnish with fresh basil leaves and serve.

Nutritional Facts (Per Serving):

Calories: 300 Protein: 28g Carbohydrates: 5g Fat: 18g

30. Salmon Salad with Cucumber and Dill

Prep Time: 10 minutes   **Cook Time: None**   **Serves: 2**

INGREDIENTS:

- 1 can wild salmon, drained
- 1/4 cup cucumber, diced
- 1 tbsp fresh dill, chopped
- 1 tbsp mayonnaise
- Salt and pepper to taste

INSTRUCTIONS:

1. In a bowl, combine salmon, cucumber, dill, and mayonnaise.
2. Season with salt and pepper.
3. Serve chilled or at room temperature.

Nutritional Facts (Per Serving):

Calories: 250 Protein: 22gCarbohydrates: 3g Fat: 17g

31. Zoodle (Zucchini Noodles) Salad with Grilled Chicken

Prep Time: 10 minutes   **Cook Time: 5 minutes**   **Serves: 2**

INGREDIENTS:

- 2 grilled chicken breasts, sliced
- 2 medium zucchinis, spiralized into noodles
- 1/4 cup cherry tomatoes, halved
- 2 tbsp pesto sauce
- Salt and pepper to taste

INSTRUCTIONS:

1. In a bowl, combine zucchini noodles, cherry tomatoes, and pesto sauce.
2. Toss to coat evenly.
3. Top with sliced grilled chicken, season with salt and pepper, and serve.

Nutritional Facts (Per Serving):

Calories: 320 Protein: 34g Carbohydrates: 8g Fat: 18g

32. Thai Chicken Lettuce Wraps

Prep Time: 10 minutes   **Cook Time: 10 minutes**   **Serves: 2**

INGREDIENTS:

- 2 grilled chicken breasts, chopped
- 4 large lettuce leaves
- 1/4 cup shredded carrots
- 1/4 cup chopped cucumber
- 2 tbsp peanut sauce (or almond butter sauce)
- 1 tbsp lime juice

INSTRUCTIONS:

1. Combine chopped chicken, shredded carrots, and cucumber in a bowl.
2. Drizzle with peanut sauce and lime juice. Mix well.
3. Spoon the mixture onto the lettuce leaves, wrap, and serve immediately.

Nutritional Facts (Per Serving):

Calories: 290 Protein: 28g Carbohydrates: 10g Fat: 16g

33. Grilled Turkey and Spinach Salad

Prep Time: 10 minutes   **Cook Time: 10 minutes**   **Serves: 2**

INGREDIENTS:

- 2 grilled turkey breasts, sliced
- 2 cups baby spinach
- 1/4 cup walnuts, chopped
- 1/4 cup feta cheese, crumbled
- 2 tbsp olive oil
- 1 tbsp balsamic vinegar

INSTRUCTIONS:

1. In a bowl, toss baby spinach, walnuts, feta cheese, olive oil, and balsamic vinegar.
2. Top with grilled turkey slices.
3. Serve immediately.

Nutritional Facts (Per Serving):

Calories: 360 Protein: 30g Carbohydrates: 8g Fat: 24g

34. Blackened Shrimp Salad

Prep Time: 5 minutes   **Cook Time: 5 minutes**   **Serves: 2**

INGREDIENTS:

- 12 shrimp, peeled and deveined
- 2 cups mixed greens
- 1 tbsp Cajun seasoning
- 1 tbsp olive oil
- 1/4 cup cherry tomatoes, halved

INSTRUCTIONS:

1. Rub Cajun seasoning onto shrimp.
2. Heat olive oil in a skillet and cook shrimp for 2-3 minutes on each side until blackened.
3. In a bowl, toss mixed greens and cherry tomatoes, and top with shrimp.
4. Serve warm.

Nutritional Facts (Per Serving):

Calories: 240 Protein: 22g Carbohydrates: 5g Fat: 15g

35. Egg Salad Lettuce Wraps

Prep Time: 10 minutes   **Cook Time: None**   **Serves: 1**

INGREDIENTS:

- 2 hard-boiled eggs, chopped
- 2 tbsp mayonnaise
- 1/4 tsp Dijon mustard
- 4 large lettuce leaves
- Salt and pepper to taste

INSTRUCTIONS:

1. In a bowl, mix chopped eggs, mayonnaise, Dijon mustard, salt, and pepper.
2. Spoon the egg salad onto the lettuce leaves and roll up.
3. Serve chilled.

Nutritional Facts (Per Serving):

Calories: 220 Protein: 12g Carbohydrates: 2g Fat: 18g

36. Turkey, Spinach, and Feta Bowl

Prep Time: 10 minutes   **Cook Time: 10 minutes**   **Serves: 2**

INGREDIENTS:

- 2 grilled turkey breasts, sliced
- 2 cups baby spinach
- 1/4 cup feta cheese, crumbled
- 1 tbsp olive oil
- 1 tbsp lemon juice
- Salt and pepper to taste

INSTRUCTIONS:

1. Heat olive oil in a pan and sauté baby spinach for 2-3 minutes until wilted.
2. Divide the spinach into bowls and top with grilled turkey and feta.
3. Drizzle with lemon juice, season with salt and pepper, and serve.

Nutritional Facts (Per Serving):

Calories: 300 Protein: 32g Carbohydrates: 6g Fat: 16g

37. Grilled Chicken Caesar Salad

Prep Time: 10 minutes   **Cook Time: 10 minutes**   **Serves: 2**

INGREDIENTS:

- 2 grilled chicken breasts, sliced
- 4 cups romaine lettuce, chopped
- 1/4 cup grated Parmesan cheese
- 2 tbsp Caesar dressing
- 1 tbsp olive oil

INSTRUCTIONS:

1. In a bowl, toss romaine lettuce with Caesar dressing and olive oil.
2. Top with grilled chicken slices and Parmesan cheese.
3. Serve immediately.

Nutritional Facts (Per Serving):

Calories: 340 Protein: 32g Carbohydrates: 4g Fat: 22g

38. Tuna and Avocado Salad

Prep Time: 5 minutes   **Cook Time: None**   **Serves: 1**

INGREDIENTS:

- 1 can tuna, drained
- 1/2 avocado, diced
- 1 tbsp olive oil
- 1 tbsp lemon juice
- Salt and pepper to taste

INSTRUCTIONS:

1. In a bowl, combine tuna, avocado, olive oil, lemon juice, salt, and pepper.
2. Serve immediately or chill for later.

Nutritional Facts (Per Serving):

Calories: 320 Protein: 22g Carbohydrates: 5g Fat: 24g

39. Turkey and Cucumber Roll-ups

Prep Time: 5 minutes   **Cook Time: None**   **Serves: 1**

INGREDIENTS:

- 4 slices deli turkey
- 4 cucumber slices
- 1 tbsp cream cheese
- Salt and pepper to taste

INSTRUCTIONS:

1. Spread cream cheese on each slice of turkey.
2. Place a cucumber slice on top, roll up, and season with salt and pepper.
3. Serve immediately.

Nutritional Facts (Per Serving):

Calories: 180 Protein: 12g Carbohydrates: 3g Fat: 14g

40. Veggie-Stuffed Chicken Breast

Prep Time: 10 minutes   **Cook Time: 25 minutes**   **Serves: 2**

INGREDIENTS:

- 2 chicken breasts, butterflied
- 1/2 cup spinach, sautéed
- 1/4 cup feta cheese, crumbled
- 1 tbsp olive oil
- Salt and pepper to taste

INSTRUCTIONS:

1. Preheat your oven to 375°F (190°C).
2. Stuff the chicken breasts with sautéed spinach and feta cheese, then secure with toothpicks.
3. Heat olive oil in a skillet and sear the chicken breasts on both sides for 3-4 minutes.
4. Transfer to a baking dish and bake for 20-25 minutes until cooked through.
5. Serve hot.

Nutritional Facts (Per Serving):

Calories: 360 Protein: 40g Carbohydrates: 2g Fat: 20g

CHAPTER 4

Dinner Recipes to Fuel Your Evenings

Dinners are where you can truly enjoy satisfying, nutrient-rich meals that don't derail your low-carb, high-protein goals. In this chapter, you'll find a variety of delicious dinner recipes that are filling and flavorful. These dishes are perfect for enjoying with family or on your own after a busy day. Each recipe is packed with lean proteins and vegetables, providing a wholesome end to your day.

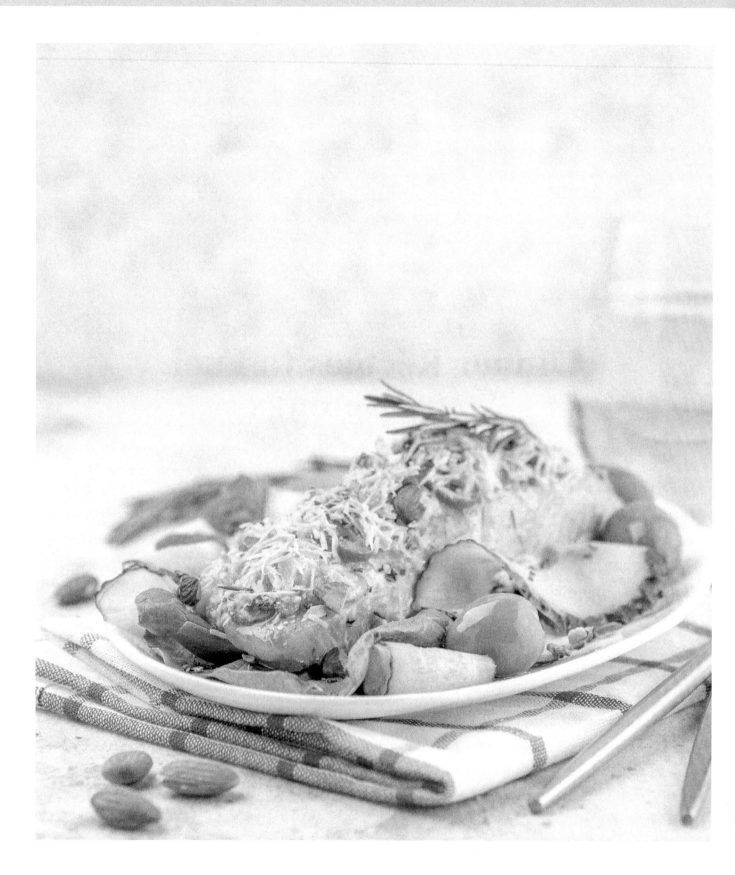

41. Grilled Lemon Garlic Salmon

Prep Time: 10 minutes   **Cook Time:** 10 minutes   **Serves:** 2

INGREDIENTS:

- 2 salmon fillets
- 1 tbsp olive oil
- 2 cloves garlic, minced
- 1 tbsp lemon juice
- Salt and pepper to taste

INSTRUCTIONS:

1. Preheat grill to medium-high heat.
2. In a small bowl, mix olive oil, garlic, and lemon juice. Brush the mixture over the salmon fillets.
3. Grill the salmon for 4-5 minutes on each side until fully cooked. Season with salt and pepper and serve hot.

Nutritional Facts (Per Serving):

Calories: 320 Protein: 34g Carbohydrates: 1g Fat: 19g

42. Low-Carb Chicken Stir-Fry

Prep Time: 10 minutes   **Cook Time:** 10 minutes   **Serves:** 2

INGREDIENTS:

- 2 boneless, skinless chicken breasts, sliced
- 1 cup broccoli florets
- 1/2 bell pepper, sliced
- 1/4 onion, sliced
- 1 tbsp soy sauce (or tamari for gluten-free)
- 1 tbsp olive oil
- 1 tsp sesame oil

INSTRUCTIONS:

1. Heat olive oil in a large pan over medium heat.
2. Add the chicken slices and cook until browned.
3. Add broccoli, bell pepper, onion, soy sauce, and sesame oil.
4. Stir-fry for 5-7 minutes until vegetables are tender. Serve hot.

Nutritional Facts (Per Serving):

Calories: 280 Protein: 36g Carbohydrates: 7g Fat: 12g

43. Baked Cod with Lemon and Herbs

Prep Time: 5 minutes   **Cook Time: 15 minutes**   **Serves: 2**

INGREDIENTS:

- 2 cod fillets
- 1 tbsp olive oil
- 1 tbsp lemon juice
- 1 tsp dried thyme
- Salt and pepper to taste

INSTRUCTIONS:

1. Preheat oven to 375°F (190°C).
2. Place cod fillets in a baking dish and drizzle with olive oil and lemon juice.
3. Sprinkle with thyme, salt, and pepper.
4. Bake for 12-15 minutes until fish is flaky. Serve with your favorite low-carb side.

Nutritional Facts (Per Serving):

Calories: 210 Protein: 34g Carbohydrates: 2g Fat: 8g

44. Chicken Parmesan (Low-Carb Version)

Prep Time: 15 minutes   **Cook Time: 20 minutes**   **Serves: 2**

INGREDIENTS:

- 2 boneless, skinless chicken breasts
- 1/4 cup almond flour
- 1/4 cup Parmesan cheese, grated
- 1/2 cup marinara sauce (sugar-free)
- 1/2 cup mozzarella cheese, shredded
- 1 tbsp olive oil
- Salt and pepper to taste

INSTRUCTIONS:

1. Preheat oven to 375°F (190°C).
2. In a bowl, mix almond flour and Parmesan cheese.
3. Coat each chicken breast with the almond flour mixture.
4. Heat olive oil in a skillet over medium heat and brown the chicken on both sides.
5. Transfer chicken to a baking dish, top with marinara sauce and mozzarella cheese, and bake for 15 minutes until the cheese is melted and bubbly.

Nutritional Facts (Per Serving):

Calories: 400 Protein: 45g Carbohydrates: 6g Fat: 22g

45. Zoodle Spaghetti with Turkey Meatballs

Prep Time: 15 minutes   **Cook Time: 15 minutes**   **Serves: 2**

INGREDIENTS:

- 2 medium zucchinis, spiralized into noodles
- 8 oz ground turkey
- 1/4 cup Parmesan cheese, grated
- 1 egg
- 1/4 cup marinara sauce (sugar-free)
- 1 tbsp olive oil
- Salt, pepper, and Italian seasoning to taste

INSTRUCTIONS:

1. Preheat oven to 375°F (190°C).
2. In a bowl, mix ground turkey, Parmesan cheese, egg, salt, pepper, and Italian seasoning.
3. Form into small meatballs and place on a baking sheet. Bake for 12-15 minutes.
4. Heat olive oil in a pan and sauté the zoodles for 3-4 minutes.
5. Top the zoodles with marinara sauce and baked turkey meatballs. Serve hot.

Nutritional Facts (Per Serving):

Calories: 350 Protein: 38g Carbohydrates: 8g Fat: 18g

46. Cauliflower Crust Pizza with Veggies

Prep Time: 15 minutes   **Cook Time: 20 minutes**   **Serves: 2**

INGREDIENTS:

- 1 small cauliflower head, grated
- 1/2 cup mozzarella cheese, shredded
- 1 egg
- 1/4 cup marinara sauce (sugar-free)
- 1/4 cup bell peppers, sliced
- 1/4 cup mushrooms, sliced
- 1 tbsp olive oil
- Salt and pepper to taste

INSTRUCTIONS:

1. Preheat oven to 400°F (200°C).
2. Steam grated cauliflower for 5-7 minutes and drain excess water.
3. In a bowl, mix cauliflower, mozzarella, egg, salt, and pepper.
4. Press the mixture onto a baking sheet lined with parchment paper to form a pizza crust.
5. Bake the crust for 10 minutes until golden.
6. Spread marinara sauce over the crust, top with bell peppers and mushrooms, and bake for another 10 minutes.

Nutritional Facts (Per Serving):

Calories: 320 Protein: 24g Carbohydrates: 10g Fat: 22g

47. Chicken and Broccoli Stir-Fry

Prep Time: 10 minutes   **Cook Time: 10 minutes**   **Serves: 2**

INGREDIENTS:

- 2 boneless, skinless chicken breasts, sliced
- 1 cup broccoli florets
- 1/4 cup onion, sliced
- 1 tbsp soy sauce (or tamari for gluten-free)
- 1 tbsp olive oil
- 1 tsp sesame oil

INSTRUCTIONS:

1. Heat olive oil in a large pan over medium heat.
2. Add the chicken slices and cook until browned.
3. Add broccoli, onion, soy sauce, and sesame oil.
4. Stir-fry for 5-7 minutes until vegetables are tender. Serve hot.

Nutritional Facts (Per Serving):

Calories: 290 Protein: 38g Carbohydrates: 6g Fat: 12g

48. Beef and Veggie Skewers

Prep Time: 15 minutes   **Cook Time: 10 minutes**   **Serves: 2**

INGREDIENTS:

- 8 oz beef sirloin, cubed
- 1/2 bell pepper, cubed
- 1/2 zucchini, sliced
- 1/2 red onion, cubed
- 1 tbsp olive oil
- 1 tsp garlic powder
- Salt and pepper to taste

INSTRUCTIONS:

1. Preheat grill to medium-high heat.
2. Thread beef, bell pepper, zucchini, and onion onto skewers.
3. Drizzle with olive oil and season with garlic powder, salt, and pepper.
4. Grill for 8-10 minutes, turning occasionally, until beef is cooked to your liking.

Nutritional Facts (Per Serving):

Calories: 350 Protein: 32g Carbohydrates: 5g Fat: 22g

49. Grilled Chicken with Avocado Salsa

Prep Time: 10 minutes   **Cook Time: 15 minutes**   **Serves: 2**

INGREDIENTS:

- 2 boneless, skinless chicken breasts
- 1 ripe avocado, diced
- 1/4 cup red onion, diced
- 1 tbsp lime juice
- 1 tbsp olive oil
- Salt and pepper to taste

INSTRUCTIONS:

1. Preheat grill to medium heat.
2. Brush chicken breasts with olive oil, season with salt and pepper, and grill for 6-8 minutes on each side until fully cooked.
3. In a bowl, combine diced avocado, red onion, lime juice, salt, and pepper.
4. Serve grilled chicken topped with avocado salsa.

Nutritional Facts (Per Serving):

Calories: 340 Protein: 40g Carbohydrates: 8g Fat: 18g

50. Eggplant Lasagna

Prep Time: 15 minutes   **Cook Time: 30 minutes**   **Serves: 2**

INGREDIENTS:

- 1 large eggplant, sliced thin
- 1/2 cup ricotta cheese
- 1/2 cup mozzarella cheese, shredded
- 1/2 cup marinara sauce (sugar-free)
- 1 tbsp olive oil
- 1 tbsp Italian seasoning
- Salt and pepper to taste

INSTRUCTIONS:

1. Preheat oven to 375°F (190°C).
2. In a baking dish, layer eggplant slices, ricotta cheese, marinara sauce, and mozzarella cheese.
3. Drizzle with olive oil and sprinkle with Italian seasoning.
4. Bake for 25-30 minutes until golden and bubbly. Serve hot.

Nutritional Facts (Per Serving):

Calories: 380 Protein: 28g Carbohydrates: 12g Fat: 25g

51. Baked Tilapia with Veggies

Prep Time: 10 minutes   **Cook Time: 20 minutes**   **Serves: 2**

INGREDIENTS:

- 2 tilapia fillets
- 1 zucchini, sliced
- 1/2 bell pepper, sliced
- 1 tbsp olive oil
- 1 tbsp lemon juice
- Salt and pepper to taste

INSTRUCTIONS:

1. Preheat the oven to 375°F (190°C).
2. Arrange tilapia fillets and veggies on a baking sheet.
3. Drizzle with olive oil and lemon juice. Season with salt and pepper.
4. Bake for 15-20 minutes, or until the tilapia is cooked through and veggies are tender.

Nutritional Facts (Per Serving):

Calories: 250 Protein: 30g Carbohydrates: 5g Fat: 12g

52. Shrimp Scampi with Zoodles

Prep Time: 10 minutes   **Cook Time: 10 minutes**   **Serves: 2**

INGREDIENTS:

- 12 shrimp, peeled and deveined
- 2 medium zucchinis, spiralized into noodles
- 2 cloves garlic, minced
- 1 tbsp butter
- 1 tbsp olive oil
- 1 tbsp lemon juice
- Salt and pepper to taste

INSTRUCTIONS:

1. Heat olive oil and butter in a skillet over medium heat.
2. Add garlic and sauté for 1 minute.
3. Add shrimp and cook for 2-3 minutes until pink.
4. Add zucchini noodles and lemon juice. Stir well and cook for an additional 2 minutes.
5. Season with salt and pepper and serve.

Nutritional Facts (Per Serving): Calories: 280 Protein: 24g Carbohydrates: 7g Fat: 18g

53. Lemon Butter Grilled Chicken

Prep Time: 10 minutes   **Cook Time: 15 minutes**   **Serves: 2**

INGREDIENTS:

- 2 boneless, skinless chicken breasts
- 1 tbsp butter
- 1 tbsp lemon juice
- 1 tsp garlic powder
- Salt and pepper to taste

INSTRUCTIONS:

1. Preheat grill to medium-high heat.
2. In a small bowl, mix melted butter, lemon juice, garlic powder, salt, and pepper.
3. Brush the mixture over the chicken breasts.
4. Grill the chicken for 6-8 minutes on each side, or until fully cooked. Serve hot.

Nutritional Facts (Per Serving):

Calories: 300 Protein: 36g Carbohydrates: 1g Fat: 16g

54. Low-Carb Chicken Alfredo

Prep Time: 10 minutes   **Cook Time: 15 minutes**   **Serves: 2**

INGREDIENTS:

- 2 boneless, skinless chicken breasts, sliced
- 1/2 cup heavy cream
- 1/4 cup Parmesan cheese, grated
- 1 tbsp butter
- 1 tsp garlic powder
- Salt and pepper to taste

INSTRUCTIONS:

1. Heat butter in a pan and cook the chicken until browned.
2. In a separate pan, heat the heavy cream and garlic powder over low heat.
3. Stir in Parmesan cheese until melted and the sauce thickens.
4. Add the cooked chicken to the Alfredo sauce and mix well.
5. Serve over your favorite low-carb pasta substitute or steamed veggies.

Nutritional Facts (Per Serving):

Calories: 450 Protein: 38g Carbohydrates: 4g Fat: 30g

55. Low-Carb Fish Tacos (Lettuce Wraps)

Prep Time: 10 minutes   **Cook Time: 10 minutes**   **Serves: 2**

INGREDIENTS:

- 2 tilapia fillets
- 4 large lettuce leaves (for wraps)
- 1/4 cup shredded cabbage
- 1/4 cup diced tomatoes
- 1 tbsp olive oil
- 1 tbsp lime juice
- Salt and pepper to taste

INSTRUCTIONS:

1. Season tilapia with salt, pepper, and lime juice.
2. Heat olive oil in a pan and cook the tilapia for 4-5 minutes on each side until flaky.
3. Place the cooked fish in lettuce leaves and top with shredded cabbage and diced tomatoes.
4. Serve immediately.

Nutritional Facts (Per Serving):

Calories: 260 Protein: 30g Carbohydrates: 5g Fat: 14g

56. Grilled Steak with Cauliflower Mash

Prep Time: 10 minutes   **Cook Time: 20 minutes**   **Serves: 2**

INGREDIENTS:

- 2 small steaks (sirloin or ribeye)
- 1 medium cauliflower head, chopped
- 1 tbsp butter
- 1 tbsp olive oil
- 1 clove garlic, minced
- Salt and pepper to taste

INSTRUCTIONS:

1. Preheat grill to medium-high heat. Season steaks with salt and pepper.
2. Grill steaks for 6-8 minutes on each side, depending on desired doneness.
3. Meanwhile, steam cauliflower until tender, then mash with butter, olive oil, and garlic. Season with salt and pepper.
4. Serve grilled steak alongside the cauliflower mash.

Nutritional Facts (Per Serving):

Calories: 450 Protein: 35g Carbohydrates: 8g Fat: 32g

57. Stir-Fried Tofu with Veggies

Prep Time: 10 minutes   **Cook Time: 10 minutes**   **Serves: 2**

INGREDIENTS:

- 1 block firm tofu, cubed
- 1 cup broccoli florets
- 1/2 bell pepper, sliced
- 1 tbsp soy sauce (or tamari for gluten-free)
- 1 tbsp olive oil
- 1 tsp sesame oil
- Salt and pepper to taste

INSTRUCTIONS:

1. Heat olive oil in a pan over medium heat.
2. Add tofu cubes and stir-fry until browned, about 5 minutes.
3. Add broccoli, bell pepper, soy sauce, sesame oil, salt, and pepper. Cook for another 5 minutes until the vegetables are tender.
4. Serve hot.

Nutritional Facts (Per Serving):

Calories: 320 Protein: 20g Carbohydrates: 7g Fat: 24g

58. Turkey-Stuffed Bell Peppers

Prep Time: 10 minutes   **Cook Time: 25 minutes**   **Serves: 2**

INGREDIENTS:

- 2 bell peppers, halved and seeds removed
- 8 oz ground turkey
- 1/4 cup diced onion
- 1/4 cup diced tomatoes
- 1/4 cup shredded cheese
- 1 tbsp olive oil
- Salt and pepper to taste

INSTRUCTIONS:

1. Preheat oven to 375°F (190°C).
2. In a pan, heat olive oil and cook the ground turkey and onions until browned.
3. Stir in diced tomatoes, salt, and pepper.
4. Stuff each bell pepper half with the turkey mixture and top with shredded cheese.
5. Bake for 20-25 minutes until the cheese is melted and peppers are tender.

Nutritional Facts (Per Serving):

Calories: 350 Protein: 28g Carbohydrates: 10g Fat: 20g

59. Garlic Butter Shrimp

Prep Time: 5 minutes   **Cook Time: 5 minutes**   **Serves: 2**

INGREDIENTS:

- 12 shrimp, peeled and deveined
- 2 tbsp butter
- 2 cloves garlic, minced
- 1 tbsp lemon juice
- Salt and pepper to taste

INSTRUCTIONS:

1. Heat butter in a skillet over medium heat.
2. Add garlic and sauté for 1 minute.
3. Add shrimp and cook for 2-3 minutes until pink.
4. Drizzle with lemon juice and season with salt and pepper. Serve hot.

Nutritional Facts (Per Serving):

Calories: 260 Protein: 24g Carbohydrates: 2g Fat: 18g

60. Low-Carb Beef and Veggie Casserole

Prep Time: 10 minutes   **Cook Time: 25 minutes**   **Serves: 4**

INGREDIENTS:

- 1 lb ground beef
- 1/2 cup diced onion
- 1/2 cup diced bell pepper
- 1/2 cup shredded cheese
- 1/2 cup cauliflower rice
- 1 tbsp olive oil
- Salt and pepper to taste

INSTRUCTIONS:

1. Preheat oven to 375°F (190°C).
2. In a pan, heat olive oil and cook the ground beef, onion, and bell pepper until the beef is browned.
3. Stir in cauliflower rice and season with salt and pepper.
4. Transfer the mixture to a baking dish and top with shredded cheese.
5. Bake for 15-20 minutes until the cheese is melted and bubbly.

Nutritional Facts (Per Serving):

Calories: 400 Protein: 30g Carbohydrates: 6g Fat: 28g

61. Creamy Spinach-Stuffed Chicken Breast

Prep Time: 10 minutes   **Cook Time: 25 minutes**   **Serves: 2**

INGREDIENTS:

- 2 boneless, skinless chicken breasts
- 1/2 cup spinach, sautéed
- 1/4 cup cream cheese
- 1/4 cup shredded mozzarella cheese
- 1 tbsp olive oil
- Salt and pepper to taste

INSTRUCTIONS:

1. Preheat oven to 375°F (190°C).
2. Cut a pocket into each chicken breast.
3. In a bowl, mix sautéed spinach, cream cheese, and mozzarella.
4. Stuff the chicken breasts with the spinach mixture and secure with toothpicks.
5. Heat olive oil in a pan and sear the chicken on both sides, then transfer to a baking dish and bake for 20-25 minutes until fully cooked.

Nutritional Facts (Per Serving):

Calories: 400 Protein: 38g Carbohydrates: 4g Fat: 26g

62. Chicken Curry with Cauliflower Rice

Prep Time: 10 minutes   **Cook Time: 20 minutes**   **Serves: 2**

INGREDIENTS:

- 2 boneless, skinless chicken breasts, cubed
- 1/2 cup coconut milk (unsweetened)
- 1 tbsp curry powder
- 1 tbsp olive oil
- 2 cups cauliflower rice
- Salt and pepper to taste

INSTRUCTIONS:

1. Heat olive oil in a pan and cook the chicken until browned.
2. Stir in curry powder and coconut milk, and simmer for 10 minutes.
3. In a separate pan, sauté cauliflower rice for 3-4 minutes.
4. Serve chicken curry over cauliflower rice.

Nutritional Facts (Per Serving):

Calories: 350 Protein: 32g Carbohydrates: 8g Fat: 22g

63. Steak Salad with Avocado

Prep Time: 10 minutes   **Cook Time: 10 minutes**   **Serves: 2**

INGREDIENTS:

- 2 small steaks (sirloin or flank)
- 4 cups mixed greens
- 1/2 avocado, sliced
- 1/4 cup cherry tomatoes, halved
- 1 tbsp olive oil
- 1 tbsp balsamic vinegar
- Salt and pepper to taste

INSTRUCTIONS:

1. Preheat grill to medium heat and grill steaks for 5-7 minutes on each side.
2. In a large bowl, toss mixed greens, avocado, cherry tomatoes, olive oil, and balsamic vinegar.
3. Slice the steaks and place on top of the salad. Serve immediately.

Nutritional Facts (Per Serving):

Calories: 400 Protein: 32g Carbohydrates: 6g Fat: 28g

64. Grilled Halibut with Asparagus

Prep Time: 10 minutes   **Cook Time: 10 minutes**   **Serves: 2**

INGREDIENTS:

- 2 halibut fillets
- 1 bunch asparagus, trimmed
- 1 tbsp olive oil
- 1 tbsp lemon juice
- Salt and pepper to taste

INSTRUCTIONS:

1. Preheat grill to medium heat.
2. Drizzle halibut and asparagus with olive oil and lemon juice, and season with salt and pepper.
3. Grill the halibut for 4-5 minutes on each side until flaky, and grill asparagus until tender.
4. Serve hot.

Nutritional Facts (Per Serving):

Calories: 320 Protein: 36g Carbohydrates: 5g Fat: 18g

65. Low-Carb Beef Stir-Fry

Prep Time: 10 minutes   **Cook Time: 10 minutes**   **Serves: 2**

INGREDIENTS:

- 8 oz beef sirloin, thinly sliced
- 1 cup broccoli florets
- 1/2 bell pepper, sliced
- 1 tbsp soy sauce (or tamari for gluten-free)
- 1 tbsp olive oil
- 1 tsp sesame oil

INSTRUCTIONS:

1. Heat olive oil in a pan over medium heat.
2. Add the beef and cook for 2-3 minutes until browned.
3. Add broccoli, bell pepper, soy sauce, and sesame oil. Stir-fry for another 5-7 minutes until the veggies are tender.
4. Serve hot.

Nutritional Facts (Per Serving):

Calories: 350 Protein: 30g Carbohydrates: 8g Fat: 22g

66. Lemon Herb Chicken Skewers

Prep Time: 10 minutes   **Cook Time: 10 minutes**   **Serves: 2**

INGREDIENTS:

- 2 boneless, skinless chicken breasts, cubed
- 1 tbsp olive oil
- 1 tbsp lemon juice
- 1 tsp dried oregano
- Salt and pepper to taste

INSTRUCTIONS:

1. Preheat grill to medium heat.
2. In a bowl, mix olive oil, lemon juice, oregano, salt, and pepper. Toss the chicken cubes in the mixture.
3. Thread the chicken onto skewers and grill for 8-10 minutes, turning occasionally.
4. Serve hot.

Nutritional Facts (Per Serving):

Calories: 280 Protein: 36g Carbohydrates: 2g Fat: 14g

67. Low-Carb Chicken Enchiladas (No Tortillas)

Prep Time: 10 minutes   **Cook Time: 20 minutes**   **Serves: 2**

INGREDIENTS:

- 2 boneless, skinless chicken breasts, shredded
- 1/2 cup enchilada sauce (sugar-free)
- 1/4 cup shredded cheese
- 1/4 cup diced green chiles
- 1 tbsp olive oil

INSTRUCTIONS:

1. Preheat oven to 375°F (190°C).
2. In a pan, heat olive oil and sauté shredded chicken with enchilada sauce and green chiles.
3. Transfer to a baking dish and top with shredded cheese.
4. Bake for 15-20 minutes until cheese is melted and bubbly.

Nutritional Facts (Per Serving):

Calories: 320 Protein: 36g Carbohydrates: 6g Fat: 18g

68. Grilled Swordfish with Garlic Butter

Prep Time: 10 minutes   **Cook Time: 10 minutes**   **Serves: 2**

INGREDIENTS:

- 2 swordfish steaks
- 2 tbsp butter
- 2 cloves garlic, minced
- 1 tbsp lemon juice
- Salt and pepper to taste

INSTRUCTIONS:

1. Preheat grill to medium heat.
2. Melt butter in a small pan, then stir in garlic and lemon juice.
3. Brush swordfish steaks with the garlic butter mixture.
4. Grill for 4-5 minutes on each side until cooked through. Serve hot.

Nutritional Facts (Per Serving):

Calories: 380 Protein: 40g Carbohydrates: 2g Fat: 22g

69. Baked Herb-Crusted Salmon

Prep Time: 10 minutes   **Cook Time: 20 minutes**   **Serves: 2**

INGREDIENTS:

- 2 salmon fillets
- 1/4 cup almond flour
- 1 tbsp fresh parsley, chopped
- 1 tbsp olive oil
- Salt and pepper to taste

INSTRUCTIONS:

1. Preheat oven to 375°F (190°C).
2. In a bowl, mix almond flour, parsley, salt, and pepper.
3. Coat each salmon fillet with the almond flour mixture and drizzle with olive oil.
4. Bake for 15-20 minutes until golden and cooked through.

Nutritional Facts (Per Serving):

Calories: 350 Protein: 34g Carbohydrates: 4g Fat: 22g

70. Grilled Chicken with Zucchini and Tomatoes

Prep Time: 10 minutes   **Cook Time: 15 minutes**   **Serves: 2**

INGREDIENTS:

- 2 boneless, skinless chicken breasts
- 1 zucchini, sliced
- 1/2 cup cherry tomatoes, halved
- 1 tbsp olive oil
- 1 tsp garlic powder
- Salt and pepper to taste

INSTRUCTIONS:

1. Preheat grill to medium heat.
2. Toss zucchini and tomatoes in olive oil, garlic powder, salt, and pepper.
3. Grill chicken breasts for 6-8 minutes on each side until fully cooked.
4. Grill zucchini and tomatoes for 4-5 minutes until tender.
5. Serve the grilled chicken with the veggies.

Nutritional Facts (Per Serving):

Calories: 320 Protein: 38g Carbohydrates: 8g Fat: 16g

CHAPTER 5

Snacks and Smoothies to Keep You on Track

When you're looking for a quick bite to boost your energy or curb cravings between meals, having healthy, high-protein snacks and smoothies on hand can make all the difference. In this chapter, you'll find easy-to-make snacks and satisfying smoothies that are perfect for keeping you on track with your low-carb, high-protein goals. Whether you're on the go or just need a little something to tide you over, these recipes will help you stay full and focused without compromising your diet.

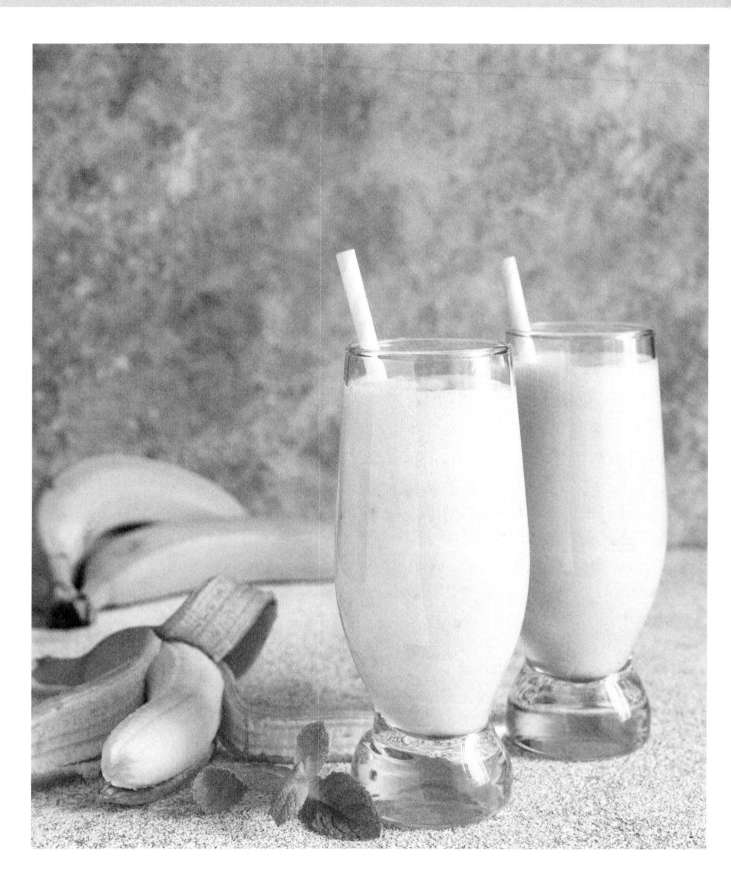

71. Almond Butter Protein Balls

Prep Time: 10 minutes   **Cook Time: None**   **Serves: 6**

INGREDIENTS:

- 1/2 cup almond butter
- 1/4 cup protein powder (vanilla or chocolate)
- 1/4 cup unsweetened shredded coconut
- 1 tbsp chia seeds
- 1 tbsp honey

INSTRUCTIONS:

1. In a bowl, mix all the ingredients until well combined.
2. Roll into small balls and refrigerate for at least 30 minutes before serving.

Nutritional Facts (Per Serving):

Calories: 120 Protein: 6g Carbohydrates: 5g Fat: 8g

72. Veggie Sticks with Hummus

Prep Time: 5 minutes   **Cook Time: None**   **Serves: 2**

INGREDIENTS:

- 1/2 cup hummus
- 1 carrot, sliced into sticks
- 1 cucumber, sliced into sticks
- 1 bell pepper, sliced into sticks

INSTRUCTIONS:

1. Arrange the veggie sticks on a plate and serve with hummus.

Nutritional Facts (Per Serving):

Calories: 150 Protein: 5g Carbohydrates: 15g Fat: 8g

73. Roasted Almonds with Sea Salt

Prep Time: 5 minutes   **Cook Time: 10 minutes**   **Serves: 4**

INGREDIENTS:

- 1 cup raw almonds
- 1 tbsp olive oil
- 1/2 tsp sea salt

INSTRUCTIONS:

1. Preheat oven to 350°F (175°C).
2. Toss the almonds with olive oil and sea salt.
3. Spread them on a baking sheet and roast for 10 minutes, stirring halfway through.

Nutritional Facts (Per Serving):

Calories: 200 Protein: 7g Carbohydrates: 6g Fat: 18g

74. Greek Yogurt with Flaxseeds

Prep Time: 5 minutes   **Cook Time: None**   **Serves: 1**

INGREDIENTS:

- 1/2 cup plain Greek yogurt
- 1 tbsp flaxseeds
- 1 tsp honey (optional)

INSTRUCTIONS:

1. Stir the flaxseeds into the yogurt and drizzle with honey, if desired.

Nutritional Facts (Per Serving):

Calories: 150 Protein: 10g Carbohydrates: 8g Fat: 7g

75. Hard-Boiled Eggs with Avocado

Prep Time: 5 minutes   **Cook Time: 10 minutes**   **Serves: 2**

INGREDIENTS:

- 2 hard-boiled eggs
- 1/2 avocado, sliced
- Salt and pepper to taste

INSTRUCTIONS:

1. Slice the hard-boiled eggs and arrange with avocado slices.
2. Season with salt and pepper and serve.

Nutritional Facts (Per Serving):

Calories: 220 Protein: 12g Carbohydrates: 4g Fat: 18g

76. Cucumber and Tuna Bites

Prep Time: 10 minutes   **Cook Time: None**   **Serves: 2**

INGREDIENTS:

- 1 can tuna, drained
- 1 tbsp mayonnaise
- 1 cucumber, sliced into rounds
- Salt and pepper to taste

INSTRUCTIONS:

1. In a bowl, mix the tuna with mayonnaise, salt, and pepper.
2. Spoon the tuna mixture onto cucumber rounds and serve.

Nutritional Facts (Per Serving):

Calories: 180 Protein: 18g Carbohydrates: 3g Fat: 10g

77. Cheese and Veggie Plate

Prep Time: 5 minutes   **Cook Time: None**   **Serves: 2**

INGREDIENTS:

- 2 oz cheddar cheese, sliced
- 1 bell pepper, sliced
- 1 carrot, sliced

INSTRUCTIONS:

1. Arrange the cheese and veggies on a plate and serve.

Nutritional Facts (Per Serving):

Calories: 200 Protein: 10g Carbohydrates: 9g Fat: 15g

78. Spicy Roasted Chickpeas

Prep Time: 5 minutes   **Cook Time: 20 minutes**   **Serves: 4**

INGREDIENTS:

- 1 can chickpeas, drained and rinsed
- 1 tbsp olive oil
- 1 tsp paprika
- 1/2 tsp cayenne pepper
- Salt to taste

INSTRUCTIONS:

1. Preheat oven to 400°F (200°C).
2. Toss chickpeas with olive oil, paprika, cayenne pepper, and salt.
3. Spread on a baking sheet and roast for 20 minutes, stirring halfway through.

Nutritional Facts (Per Serving):

Calories: 150 Protein: 7g Carbohydrates: 20g Fat: 6g

79. Protein-Packed Smoothie (Vanilla Almond)

Prep Time: 5 minutes   **Cook Time: None**   **Serves: 1**

INGREDIENTS:

- 1 scoop vanilla protein powder
- 1 cup unsweetened almond milk
- 1 tbsp almond butter
- 1/2 tsp vanilla extract

INSTRUCTIONS:

1. Blend all ingredients together until smooth. Serve immediately.

Nutritional Facts (Per Serving):

Calories: 200 Protein: 20g Carbohydrates: 6g Fat: 12g

80. Berry Blast Smoothie

Prep Time: 5 minutes   **Cook Time: None**   **Serves: 1**

INGREDIENTS:

- 1/2 cup mixed berries (strawberries, blueberries, raspberries)
- 1 scoop vanilla protein powder
- 1/2 cup unsweetened almond milk
- 1/4 cup ice cubes

INSTRUCTIONS:

1. Blend all ingredients until smooth. Serve immediately.

Nutritional Facts (Per Serving):

Calories: 160 Protein: 18g Carbohydrates: 12g Fat: 5g

81. Green Power Smoothie

Prep Time: 5 minutes   **Cook Time: None**   **Serves: 1**

INGREDIENTS:

- 1/2 cup spinach
- 1/4 avocado
- 1/2 cup unsweetened almond milk
- 1 scoop vanilla protein powder

INSTRUCTIONS:

1. Blend all ingredients until smooth. Serve immediately.

Nutritional Facts (Per Serving):

Calories: 160 Protein: 18g Carbohydrates: 5g Fat: 8g

82. Chocolate Peanut Butter Smoothie

Prep Time: 5 minutes   **Cook Time: None**   **Serves: 1**

INGREDIENTS:

- 1 scoop chocolate protein powder
- 1 tbsp peanut butter
- 1/2 cup unsweetened almond milk
- 1/4 cup ice cubes

INSTRUCTIONS:

1. Blend all ingredients together until smooth. Serve immediately.

Nutritional Facts (Per Serving):

Calories: 250 Protein: 20g Carbohydrates: 6g Fat: 16g

83. Avocado Spinach Smoothie

Prep Time: 5 minutes   **Cook Time: None**   **Serves: 1**

INGREDIENTS:

- 1/2 avocado
- 1/2 cup spinach
- 1/2 cup unsweetened almond milk
- 1 tbsp chia seeds

INSTRUCTIONS:

1. Blend all ingredients until smooth. Serve immediately.

Nutritional Facts (Per Serving):

Calories: 220 Protein: 8g Carbohydrates: 7g Fat: 18g

84. Tropical Mango Smoothie

Prep Time: 5 minutes   **Cook Time: None**   **Serves: 1**

INGREDIENTS:

- 1/4 cup frozen mango
- 1/2 cup unsweetened coconut milk
- 1 scoop vanilla protein powder
- 1/4 cup ice cubes

INSTRUCTIONS:

1. Blend all ingredients until smooth. Serve immediately.

Nutritional Facts (Per Serving):

Calories: 180 Protein: 18g Carbohydrates: 10g Fat: 8g

85. Blueberry and Kale Smoothie

Prep Time: 5 minutes   **Cook Time: None**   **Serves: 1**

INGREDIENTS:

- 1/2 cup frozen blueberries
- 1/2 cup kale
- 1 scoop vanilla protein powder
- 1/2 cup unsweetened almond milk

INSTRUCTIONS:

1. Blend all ingredients together until smooth. Serve immediately.

Nutritional Facts (Per Serving):

Calories: 160 Protein: 18g Carbohydrates: 10g Fat: 5g

86. Matcha Protein Smoothie

Prep Time: 5 minutes   **Cook Time: None**   **Serves: 1**

INGREDIENTS:

- 1 scoop vanilla protein powder
- 1/2 tsp matcha powder
- 1/2 cup unsweetened almond milk
- 1/4 cup ice cubes

INSTRUCTIONS:

1. Blend all ingredients together until smooth. Serve immediately.

Nutritional Facts (Per Serving):

Calories: 150 Protein: 18g Carbohydrates: 4g Fat: 5g

87. Strawberry Banana Protein Shake

Prep Time: 5 minutes   **Cook Time: None**   **Serves: 1**

INGREDIENTS:

- 1/2 banana
- 1/4 cup strawberries
- 1 scoop vanilla protein powder
- 1/2 cup unsweetened almond milk

INSTRUCTIONS:

1. Blend all ingredients together until smooth. Serve immediately.

Nutritional Facts (Per Serving):

Calories: 180 Protein: 18g Carbohydrates: 20g Fat: 4g

88. Chocolate Coconut Smoothie

Prep Time: 5 minutes   **Cook Time: None**   **Serves: 1**

INGREDIENTS:

- 1 scoop chocolate protein powder
- 1/2 cup coconut milk (unsweetened)
- 1 tbsp shredded unsweetened coconut
- 1/4 cup ice cubes

INSTRUCTIONS:

1. Blend all ingredients until smooth. Serve immediately.

Nutritional Facts (Per Serving):

Calories: 220 Protein: 20g Carbohydrates: 6g Fat: 15g

89. Almond and Spinach Smoothie

Prep Time: 5 minutes   **Cook Time: None**   **Serves: 1**

INGREDIENTS:

- 1/4 cup almond butter
- 1/2 cup spinach
- 1 scoop vanilla protein powder
- 1/2 cup unsweetened almond milk

INSTRUCTIONS:

1. Blend all ingredients until smooth. Serve immediately.

Nutritional Facts (Per Serving):

Calories: 250 Protein: 18g Carbohydrates: 8g Fat: 18g

90. Raspberry Chia Pudding

**Prep Time: 10 minutes
(plus chilling time)**   **Cook Time: None**   **Serves: 2**

INGREDIENTS:

- 1/4 cup chia seeds
- 1 cup unsweetened almond milk
- 1/4 cup fresh raspberries
- 1 tsp vanilla extract

INSTRUCTIONS:

1. Mix chia seeds, almond milk, and vanilla extract in a bowl.
2. Let it sit for at least 2 hours or overnight in the refrigerator.
3. Top with fresh raspberries before serving.

Nutritional Facts (Per Serving):

Calories: 160 Protein: 6g Carbohydrates: 8g Fat: 12g

91. Turkey Roll-Ups with Cream Cheese

Prep Time: 5 minutes   **Cook Time: None**   **Serves: 1**

INGREDIENTS:

- 2 slices deli turkey
- 1 tbsp cream cheese
- 1/4 cucumber, sliced into thin strips

INSTRUCTIONS:

1. Spread cream cheese on the turkey slices.
2. Add cucumber slices and roll up tightly.
3. Secure with a toothpick if necessary and serve.

Nutritional Facts (Per Serving):

Calories: 150 Protein: 12g Carbohydrates: 2g Fat: 10g

92. Celery Sticks with Almond Butter

Prep Time: 5 minutes   **Cook Time: None**   **Serves: 1**

INGREDIENTS:

- 2 celery sticks
- 2 tbsp almond butter

INSTRUCTIONS:

1. Spread almond butter onto the celery sticks and serve.

Nutritional Facts (Per Serving):

Calories: 190 Protein: 7g Carbohydrates: 6g Fat: 16g

93. Sunflower Seeds with Hard-Boiled Egg

Prep Time: 5 minutes   **Cook Time: None**   **Serves: 1**

INGREDIENTS:

- 1 hard-boiled egg
- 1/4 cup sunflower seeds

INSTRUCTIONS:

1. Serve the hard-boiled egg alongside a handful of sunflower seeds.

Nutritional Facts (Per Serving):

Calories: 220 Protein: 12g Carbohydrates: 4g Fat: 18g

94. Almond Flour Crackers with Guacamole

Prep Time: 10 minutes   **Cook Time: None**   **Serves: 2**

INGREDIENTS:

- 1/2 cup almond flour crackers (store-bought or homemade)
- 1/4 cup guacamole

INSTRUCTIONS:

1. Serve the almond flour crackers with guacamole as a dip.

Nutritional Facts (Per Serving):

Calories: 180 Protein: 6g Carbohydrates: 8g Fat: 14g

95. Cottage Cheese with Cucumber Slices

Prep Time: 5 minutes   **Cook Time: None**   **Serves: 1**

INGREDIENTS:

- 1/2 cup cottage cheese
- 1/4 cucumber, sliced

INSTRUCTIONS:

1. Serve the cottage cheese with cucumber slices on the side.

Nutritional Facts (Per Serving):

Calories: 140 Protein: 12g Carbohydrates: 4g Fat: 8g

96. Protein Bars (Homemade)

Prep Time: 10 minutes   **Cook Time: None**   **Serves: 6**

INGREDIENTS:

- 1 cup protein powder (vanilla or chocolate)
- 1/2 cup almond butter
- 1/4 cup unsweetened coconut flakes
- 2 tbsp honey

INSTRUCTIONS:

1. In a bowl, mix all ingredients until well combined.
2. Press into a baking dish and refrigerate for 1 hour before cutting into bars.

Nutritional Facts (Per Serving):

Calories: 200 Protein: 15g Carbohydrates: 8g Fat: 12g

97. Roasted Pumpkin Seeds

Prep Time: 5 minutes **Cook Time: 15 minutes** **Serves: 4**

INGREDIENTS:

- 1 cup pumpkin seeds
- 1 tbsp olive oil
- 1/2 tsp salt

INSTRUCTIONS:

1. Preheat the oven to 350°F (175°C).
2. Toss pumpkin seeds with olive oil and salt.
3. Spread on a baking sheet and roast for 12-15 minutes, stirring halfway through.

Nutritional Facts (Per Serving):

Calories: 150 Protein: 7g Carbohydrates: 5g Fat: 12g

98. Greek Yogurt and Berry Smoothie

Prep Time: 5 minutes **Cook Time: None** **Serves: 1**

INGREDIENTS:

- 1/2 cup plain Greek yogurt
- 1/4 cup mixed berries (frozen or fresh)
- 1/2 cup unsweetened almond milk

INSTRUCTIONS:

1. Blend all ingredients together until smooth. Serve immediately.

Nutritional Facts (Per Serving):

Calories: 160 Protein: 14g Carbohydrates: 10g Fat: 6g

99. Low-Carb Lemon Bars

Prep Time: 10 minutes   **Cook Time: 20 minutes**   **Serves: 8**

INGREDIENTS:

- 1 cup almond flour
- 1/4 cup butter, melted
- 1/4 cup lemon juice
- 2 eggs
- 1/4 cup sweetener (erythritol or monk fruit)

INSTRUCTIONS:

1. Preheat oven to 350°F (175°C).
2. In a bowl, mix almond flour and melted butter to form a crust and press into a baking dish.
3. Bake the crust for 10 minutes.
4. In a separate bowl, whisk together lemon juice, eggs, and sweetener.
5. Pour the lemon mixture over the crust and bake for another 10 minutes. Let cool before serving.

Nutritional Facts (Per Serving):

Calories: 150 Protein: 5g Carbohydrates: 4g Fat: 12g

100. Almond Flour Blueberry Muffin

Prep Time: 10 minutes   **Cook Time: 20 minutes**   **Serves: 6**

INGREDIENTS:

- 1 cup almond flour
- 1/4 cup blueberries
- 2 eggs
- 1/4 cup almond milk
- 1 tsp baking powder
- 1/4 cup sweetener (erythritol or monk fruit)

INSTRUCTIONS:

1. Preheat oven to 350°F (175°C).
2. In a bowl, whisk eggs, almond milk, and sweetener.
3. Stir in almond flour and baking powder, then gently fold in blueberries.
4. Pour the batter into muffin molds and bake for 20 minutes.

Nutritional Facts (Per Serving):

Calories: 180 Protein: 7g Carbohydrates: 6g Fat: 14g

CHAPTER 6

The 60-Day Meal Plan:
A Step-by-Step Guide

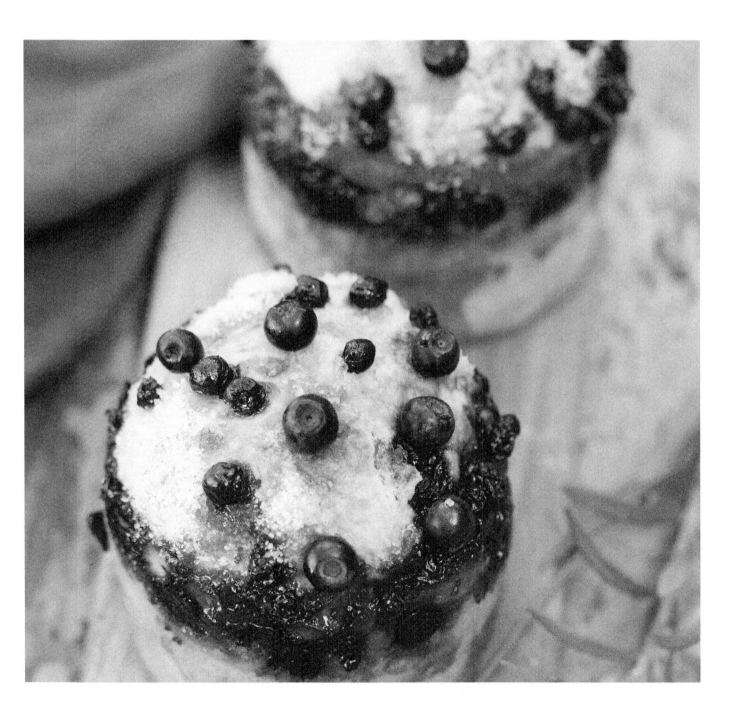

Embarking on a 60-day meal plan can seem daunting, but it doesn't have to be. With the right strategy, this plan is designed to integrate seamlessly into your lifestyle, offering flexible options that fit your schedule while delivering sustainable results. The 60-day meal plan is a practical guide that helps you stay on track, improve your eating habits, and achieve your weight loss and strength-building goals without unnecessary stress. This chapter will walk you through how to use the plan, prep your meals, and make necessary adjustments as you progress.

How to Use the 60-Day Meal Plan

The 60-day meal plan is designed to guide you through two months of balanced, high-protein, low-carb eating that will help you shed fat while maintaining or building muscle. The plan incorporates a variety of meals to keep you engaged and satisfied, and it's structured to offer both simplicity and flexibility.

To begin, each week is broken down into daily meals, including breakfast, lunch, dinner, and snacks. These meals are pre-planned to ensure that you stay within your nutritional targets, particularly in keeping carbs low while maintaining high protein levels. As you move through the plan, feel free to swap out meals that better fit your preferences or adjust portions based on your progress and needs.

The meal plan isn't restrictive but rather a tool that helps you stay consistent. If you're short on time one day, you'll find quick-prep meals that still hit your macros. On days when you have more time, you can experiment with new recipes from the plan. Remember, the key is consistency and balance, not perfection.

Weekly Meal Prep Tips for Success

Meal prepping is one of the most effective ways to ensure success on a structured meal plan. It helps you save time, stay organized, and avoid unhealthy food choices when you're in a rush or feeling tired. Here are a few tips to make weekly meal prep more manageable:

1. **Choose a Prep Day**: Set aside a specific day of the week for meal prepping, such as Sunday. This will allow you to prepare meals for the next few days in advance, reducing the need to cook daily.

2. **Batch Cook Proteins**: Cook larger quantities of staple proteins such as grilled chicken, ground turkey, or salmon. These proteins can be stored in the fridge and used in different meals throughout the week, whether in salads, wraps, or bowls.

3. **Prepare Your Veggies**: Pre-chop vegetables like bell peppers, cucumbers, zucchini, and leafy greens so they are ready to go. Store them in airtight containers for easy access when making salads, stir-fries, or snacks.

4. **Plan Snacks**: Have your snacks ready to grab and go. Portion out almonds, protein bars, or boiled eggs in small containers, so you're never left reaching for unhealthy options.

5. **Store and Label**: Use clear, labeled containers to store your meals. This helps you see what's available at a glance and prevents any confusion or waste.

By prepping ahead, you eliminate the daily stress of figuring out what to eat, allowing you to focus on other important aspects of your day.

Flexible Recipes for Different Days

The beauty of this meal plan is its flexibility. While the plan provides specific meal suggestions for each day, it's designed for you to swap out recipes based on what you feel like eating or what ingredients you have on hand. Here are a few ideas to keep your meals varied without straying from your nutritional goals:

1. **Swap Proteins**: If a recipe calls for chicken but you prefer turkey or fish

that day, feel free to switch them. The goal is to keep the protein content high, so as long as you stay within similar portions, you're on track.

2. **Mix and Match Vegetables**: Don't feel confined to the specific vegetables listed in a recipe. Substitute with what's fresh or available—zucchini instead of broccoli, spinach instead of kale. The key is to maintain a balance of fiber-rich vegetables in your meals.

3. **Switch Up Your Snacks**: If you're tired of eating the same snack every day, swap in one of the other snack recipes from Chapter 5. For example, if you had cheese and veggie sticks earlier in the week, try protein balls or hard-boiled eggs the next time.

4. **Use Leftovers Wisely**: Leftovers are a great way to save time and reduce food waste. If you have leftover grilled chicken from dinner, use it in a salad or wrap for lunch the next day. Similarly, leftover veggies can be added to omelets or stir-fries.

These flexible options keep the plan from feeling restrictive, allowing you to enjoy a variety of flavors while staying consistent with your goals.

Adjusting the Meal Plan for Results

As you progress through the 60-day meal plan, you may find that adjustments are necessary depending on your individual results and lifestyle changes. Here are some ways you can adjust the plan to continue seeing results:

1. **Monitor Portion Sizes**: If you're not losing weight or seeing the desired changes in muscle tone, it might be time to adjust your portion sizes. Reducing carb portions slightly or increasing protein can help improve results. However, avoid making drastic changes—small adjustments over time are more effective.

2. **Increase Physical Activity**: The meal plan works best when paired with regular physical activity. If your primary goal is to build muscle, make sure you're incorporating strength training into your routine. If weight loss is your focus, adding cardio can boost results.

3. **Tailor to Your Schedule**: If you have particularly busy weeks, consider prepping more "grab-and-go" meals and snacks to stay on track. Conversely, if you have more free time, you might want to experiment with new recipes and meal variations.

4. **Adjust for Dietary Needs**: If you develop new dietary preferences or sensitivities, such as dairy-free or gluten-free needs, adjust your recipes accordingly. There are plenty of low-carb, high-protein alternatives available to ensure you still hit your nutritional targets.

By monitoring your progress and making thoughtful adjustments, you'll ensure that the plan continues working for you throughout the 60 days.

Tips for Staying Consistent with the Plan

Staying consistent with any meal plan requires a mix of discipline, flexibility, and support. Here are a few tips to help you stay on track for the full 60 days:

1. **Set Short-Term Goals**: Breaking the 60-day plan into smaller, more manageable chunks can make it feel less overwhelming. Set weekly or bi-weekly goals and celebrate small victories like sticking to your prep days or avoiding sugar for the week.

2. **Stay Hydrated**: Drinking plenty of water is key to both fat loss and muscle building. Staying hydrated helps you feel full and energized, reducing cravings for unhealthy snacks.

3. **Don't Deprive Yourself**: If you find yourself craving something outside of the plan, it's okay to indulge occasionally. The key is moderation—enjoying a treat once in a while can keep you from feeling deprived and help you stay on track in the long run.

4. **Find a Support System**: Having a friend, family member, or online community to share your progress and challenges with can make all the difference. Accountability partners can help keep you motivated, share meal ideas, and celebrate successes with you.

5. **Track Your Progress**: Keeping a food journal or using a meal-tracking app

can help you stay mindful of what you're eating and how it aligns with your goals. It also allows you to look back and see how far you've come, which can be incredibly motivating.

By following these tips and staying focused on your long-term goals, you'll be well on your way to completing the 60-day meal plan and achieving lasting success.

CHAPTER 7

Meal Plans for Weight Loss and Strength Building

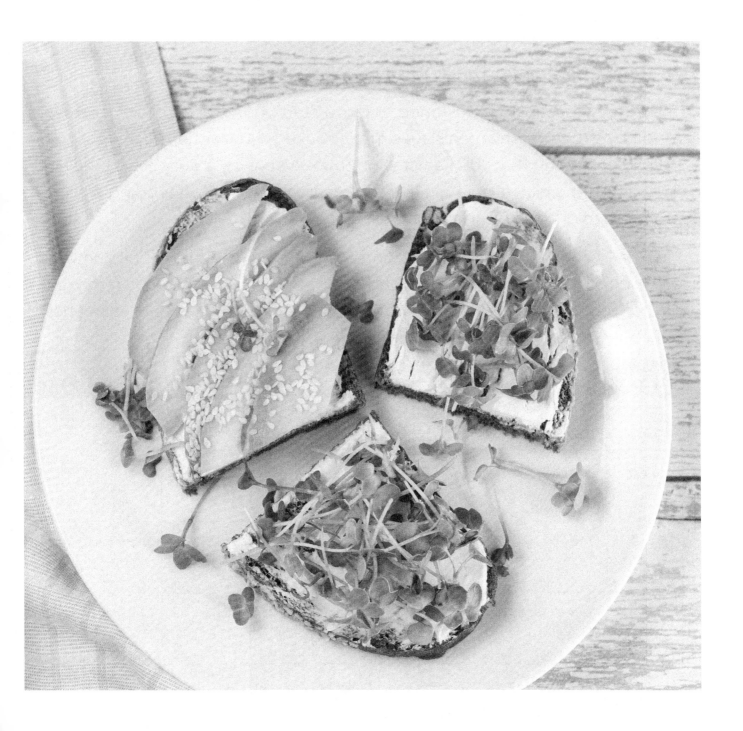

This chapter introduces two structured meal plans designed to help you achieve your weight loss and muscle-building goals. Whether you're seeking quick results in 28 days or looking for a more sustainable approach with a 60-day plan, these meal plans offer simplicity, flexibility, and a balanced approach to nutrition. With a focus on high-protein, low-carb meals, you'll stay satisfied, energized, and motivated as you work toward your goals.

28-Day Meal Plan for Quick Results

The 28-day meal plan is designed to jump-start your progress with an easy-to-follow structure. The meals are simple, packed with nutrients, and quick to prepare, ensuring that you can stay on track even with a busy schedule. The flexibility of the plan allows you to swap meals as needed, depending on your preferences or available ingredients.

Each day includes breakfast, lunch, dinner, and snacks, with the recipe numbers corresponding to those found in previous chapters. Follow the plan day-by-day for best results, and feel free to experiment with meal swaps as needed to keep things fresh.

DAY	BREAKFAST	LUNCH	DINNER	SNACK
Day 1	1. Classic Protein Omelette	5. Low-Carb Cobb Salad	41. Grilled Lemon Garlic Salmon	71. Almond Butter Protein Balls
Day 2	3. Avocado and Egg Bowl	7. Tuna Salad Lettuce Wraps	44. Chicken Parmesan (Low-Carb Version)	73. Roasted Almonds with Sea Salt
Day 3	9. Low-Carb Breakfast Burrito	11. Grilled Lemon Garlic Chicken Salad	46. Cauliflower Crust Pizza with Veggies	75. Hard-Boiled Eggs with Avocado
Day 4	5. Greek Yogurt Protein Parfait	12. Turkey and Cheese Breakfast Wrap	48. Beef and Veggie Skewers	76. Cucumber and Tuna Bites

DAY	BREAKFAST	LUNCH	DINNER	SNACK
Day 5	6. Almond Flour Pancakes	14. Zucchini Fritters with Egg	51. Baked Tilapia with Veggies	77. Cheese and Veggie Plate
Day 6	10. Chia Seed Pudding with Berries	18. Thai Chicken Lettuce Wraps	53. Lemon Butter Grilled Chicken	79. Protein-Packed Smoothie (Vanilla Almond)
Day 7	13. Low-Carb Granola with Nuts and Seeds	21. Greek Chicken Salad with Feta	56. Grilled Steak with Cauliflower Mash	81. Green Power Smoothie
Day 8	8. Spinach and Feta Frittata	16. Caprese Salad with Chicken	57. Stir-Fried Tofu with Veggies	83. Avocado Spinach Smoothie
Day 9	4. Egg Muffins with Veggies	10. Cauliflower Rice with Grilled Chicken	60. Low-Carb Beef and Veggie Casserole	84. Tropical Mango Smoothie
Day 10	2. Low-Carb Breakfast Casserole	15. Salmon Salad with Cucumber and Dill	62. Chicken Curry with Cauliflower Rice	85. Blueberry and Kale Smoothie
Day 11	12. Turkey and Cheese Breakfast Wrap	19. Grilled Turkey and Spinach Salad	63. Steak Salad with Avocado	90. Raspberry Chia Pudding
Day 12	7. Smoked Salmon & Cream Cheese Roll	17. Zoodle Salad with Grilled Chicken	65. Low-Carb Beef Stir-Fry	92. Celery Sticks with Almond Butter
Day 13	14. Zucchini Fritters with Egg	22. Shrimp and Avocado Salad	66. Lemon Herb Chicken Skewers	94. Almond Flour Crackers with Guacamole
Day 14	11. Grilled Lemon Garlic Chicken Salad	24. Mediterranean Chickpea Salad (Low-Carb)	67. Low-Carb Chicken Enchiladas (No Tortillas)	96. Protein Bars (Homemade)
Day 15	15. Cottage Cheese and Berry Bowl	25. Grilled Chicken Caesar Salad	68. Grilled Swordfish with Garlic Butter	97. Roasted Pumpkin Seeds
Day 16	9. Low-Carb Breakfast Burrito	23. Turkey and Veggie Roll-ups	69. Baked Herb-Crusted Salmon	99. Low-Carb Lemon Bars

DAY	BREAKFAST	LUNCH	DINNER	SNACK
Day 17	13. Low-Carb Granola with Nuts and Seeds	26. Tuna and Avocado Salad	70. Grilled Chicken with Zucchini and Tomatoes	100. Almond Flour Blueberry Muffin
Day 18	1. Classic Protein Omelette	8. Spinach and Feta Frittata	52. Shrimp Scampi with Zoodles	91. Turkey Roll-Ups with Cream Cheese
Day 19	5. Greek Yogurt Protein Parfait	9. Low-Carb Breakfast Burrito	55. Low-Carb Fish Tacos (Lettuce Wraps)	76. Cucumber and Tuna Bites
Day 20	2. Low-Carb Breakfast Casserole	13. Low-Carb Granola with Nuts and Seeds	54. Low-Carb Chicken Alfredo	95. Cottage Cheese with Cucumber Slices
Day 21	14. Zucchini Fritters with Egg	17. Zoodle Salad with Grilled Chicken	59. Garlic Butter Shrimp	93. Sunflower Seeds with Hard-Boiled Egg
Day 22	7. Smoked Salmon & Cream Cheese Roll	16. Caprese Salad with Chicken	64. Grilled Halibut with Asparagus	89. Almond and Spinach Smoothie
Day 23	3. Avocado and Egg Bowl	10. Cauliflower Rice with Grilled Chicken	43. Baked Cod with Lemon and Herbs	79. Protein-Packed Smoothie (Vanilla Almond)
Day 24	4. Egg Muffins with Veggies	18. Thai Chicken Lettuce Wraps	61. Creamy Spinach-Stuffed Chicken Breast	85. Blueberry and Kale Smoothie
Day 25	6. Almond Flour Pancakes	19. Grilled Turkey and Spinach Salad	45. Zoodle Spaghetti with Turkey Meatballs	82. Chocolate Peanut Butter Smoothie
Day 26	15. Cottage Cheese and Berry Bowl	24. Mediterranean Chickpea Salad (Low-Carb)	53. Lemon Butter Grilled Chicken	87. Strawberry Banana Protein Shake
Day 27	12. Turkey and Cheese Breakfast Wrap	25. Grilled Chicken Caesar Salad	49. Grilled Chicken with Avocado Salsa	96. Protein Bars (Homemade)

DAY	BREAKFAST	LUNCH	DINNER	SNACK
Day 28	10. Chia Seed Pudding with Berries	14. Zucchini Fritters with Egg	50. Eggplant Lasagna	84. Tropical Mango Smoothie

60-Day Flexible Meal Plan for Lasting Success

This 60-day meal plan provides a long-term approach to weight loss and muscle-building. Like the 28-day plan, it focuses on high-protein, low-carb meals to help you stay satisfied and energized while making progress toward your goals. Each day features recipes from earlier chapters, with flexibility to swap meals and adjust portions based on your needs.

DAY	BREAKFAST	LUNCH	DINNER	SNACK
Day 1	1. Classic Protein Omelette	5. Low-Carb Cobb Salad	41. Grilled Lemon Garlic Salmon	71. Almond Butter Protein Balls
Day 2	3. Avocado and Egg Bowl	7. Tuna Salad Lettuce Wraps	44. Chicken Parmesan (Low-Carb Version)	73. Roasted Almonds with Sea Salt
Day 3	9. Low-Carb Breakfast Burrito	11. Grilled Lemon Garlic Chicken Salad	46. Cauliflower Crust Pizza with Veggies	75. Hard-Boiled Eggs with Avocado
Day 4	5. Greek Yogurt Protein Parfait	12. Turkey and Cheese Breakfast Wrap	48. Beef and Veggie Skewers	76. Cucumber and Tuna Bites
Day 5	6. Almond Flour Pancakes	14. Zucchini Fritters with Egg	51. Baked Tilapia with Veggies	77. Cheese and Veggie Plate
Day 6	10. Chia Seed Pudding with Berries	18. Thai Chicken Lettuce Wraps	53. Lemon Butter Grilled Chicken	79. Protein-Packed Smoothie (Vanilla Almond)
Day 7	13. Low-Carb Granola with Nuts and Seeds	21. Greek Chicken Salad with Feta	56. Grilled Steak with Cauliflower Mash	81. Green Power Smoothie

DAY	BREAKFAST	LUNCH	DINNER	SNACK
Day 8	8. Spinach and Feta Frittata	16. Caprese Salad with Chicken	57. Stir-Fried Tofu with Veggies	83. Avocado Spinach Smoothie
Day 9	4. Egg Muffins with Veggies	10. Cauliflower Rice with Grilled Chicken	60. Low-Carb Beef and Veggie Casserole	84. Tropical Mango Smoothie
Day 10	2. Low-Carb Breakfast Casserole	15. Salmon Salad with Cucumber and Dill	62. Chicken Curry with Cauliflower Rice	85. Blueberry and Kale Smoothie
Day 11	12. Turkey and Cheese Breakfast Wrap	19. Grilled Turkey and Spinach Salad	63. Steak Salad with Avocado	90. Raspberry Chia Pudding
Day 12	7. Smoked Salmon & Cream Cheese Roll	17. Zoodle Salad with Grilled Chicken	65. Low-Carb Beef Stir-Fry	92. Celery Sticks with Almond Butter
Day 13	14. Zucchini Fritters with Egg	22. Shrimp and Avocado Salad	66. Lemon Herb Chicken Skewers	94. Almond Flour Crackers with Guacamole
Day 14	11. Grilled Lemon Garlic Chicken Salad	24. Mediterranean Chickpea Salad (Low-Carb)	67. Low-Carb Chicken Enchiladas (No Tortillas)	96. Protein Bars (Homemade)
Day 15	15. Cottage Cheese and Berry Bowl	25. Grilled Chicken Caesar Salad	68. Grilled Swordfish with Garlic Butter	97. Roasted Pumpkin Seeds
Day 16	9. Low-Carb Breakfast Burrito	23. Turkey and Veggie Roll-ups	69. Baked Herb-Crusted Salmon	99. Low-Carb Lemon Bars
Day 17	13. Low-Carb Granola with Nuts and Seeds	26. Tuna and Avocado Salad	70. Grilled Chicken with Zucchini and Tomatoes	100. Almond Flour Blueberry Muffin
Day 18	1. Classic Protein Omelette	8. Spinach and Feta Frittata	52. Shrimp Scampi with Zoodles	91. Turkey Roll-Ups with Cream Cheese
Day 19	5. Greek Yogurt Protein Parfait	9. Low-Carb Breakfast Burrito	55. Low-Carb Fish Tacos (Lettuce Wraps)	76. Cucumber and Tuna Bites

DAY	BREAKFAST	LUNCH	DINNER	SNACK
Day 20	2. Low-Carb Breakfast Casserole	13. Low-Carb Granola with Nuts and Seeds	54. Low-Carb Chicken Alfredo	95. Cottage Cheese with Cucumber Slices
Day 21	14. Zucchini Fritters with Egg	17. Zoodle Salad with Grilled Chicken	59. Garlic Butter Shrimp	93. Sunflower Seeds with Hard-Boiled Egg
Day 22	7. Smoked Salmon & Cream Cheese Roll	16. Caprese Salad with Chicken	64. Grilled Halibut with Asparagus	89. Almond and Spinach Smoothie
Day 23	3. Avocado and Egg Bowl	10. Cauliflower Rice with Grilled Chicken	43. Baked Cod with Lemon and Herbs	79. Protein-Packed Smoothie (Vanilla Almond)
Day 24	4. Egg Muffins with Veggies	18. Thai Chicken Lettuce Wraps	61. Creamy Spinach-Stuffed Chicken Breast	85. Blueberry and Kale Smoothie
Day 25	6. Almond Flour Pancakes	19. Grilled Turkey and Spinach Salad	45. Zoodle Spaghetti with Turkey Meatballs	82. Chocolate Peanut Butter Smoothie
Day 26	15. Cottage Cheese and Berry Bowl	24. Mediterranean Chickpea Salad (Low-Carb)	53. Lemon Butter Grilled Chicken	87. Strawberry Banana Protein Shake
Day 27	12. Turkey and Cheese Breakfast Wrap	25. Grilled Chicken Caesar Salad	49. Grilled Chicken with Avocado Salsa	96. Protein Bars (Homemade)
Day 28	10. Chia Seed Pudding with Berries	14. Zucchini Fritters with Egg	50. Eggplant Lasagna	84. Tropical Mango Smoothie
Day 29	5. Greek Yogurt Protein Parfait	7. Tuna Salad Lettuce Wraps	41. Grilled Lemon Garlic Salmon	71. Almond Butter Protein Balls
Day 30	9. Low-Carb Breakfast Burrito	16. Caprese Salad with Chicken	46. Cauliflower Crust Pizza with Veggies	75. Hard-Boiled Eggs with Avocado

DAY	BREAKFAST	LUNCH	DINNER	SNACK
Day 31	6. Almond Flour Pancakes	8. Spinach and Feta Frittata	48. Beef and Veggie Skewers	71. Almond Butter Protein Balls
Day 32	1. Classic Protein Omelette	10. Cauliflower Rice with Grilled Chicken	53. Lemon Butter Grilled Chicken	73. Roasted Almonds with Sea Salt
Day 33	9. Low-Carb Breakfast Burrito	21. Greek Chicken Salad with Feta	46. Cauliflower Crust Pizza with Veggies	75. Hard-Boiled Eggs with Avocado
Day 34	5. Greek Yogurt Protein Parfait	12. Turkey and Cheese Breakfast Wrap	44. Chicken Parmesan (Low-Carb Version)	77. Cheese and Veggie Plate
Day 35	7. Smoked Salmon & Cream Cheese Roll	11. Grilled Lemon Garlic Chicken Salad	41. Grilled Lemon Garlic Salmon	79. Protein-Packed Smoothie (Vanilla Almond)
Day 36	4. Egg Muffins with Veggies	13. Low-Carb Granola with Nuts and Seeds	49. Grilled Chicken with Avocado Salsa	81. Green Power Smoothie
Day 37	2. Low-Carb Breakfast Casserole	16. Caprese Salad with Chicken	43. Baked Cod with Lemon and Herbs	83. Avocado Spinach Smoothie
Day 38	14. Zucchini Fritters with Egg	22. Shrimp and Avocado Salad	55. Low-Carb Fish Tacos (Lettuce Wraps)	85. Blueberry and Kale Smoothie
Day 39	3. Avocado and Egg Bowl	24. Mediterranean Chickpea Salad (Low-Carb)	59. Garlic Butter Shrimp	87. Strawberry Banana Protein Shake
Day 40	10. Chia Seed Pudding with Berries	17. Zoodle Salad with Grilled Chicken	60. Low-Carb Beef and Veggie Casserole	89. Almond and Spinach Smoothie
Day 41	12. Turkey and Cheese Breakfast Wrap	25. Grilled Chicken Caesar Salad	62. Chicken Curry with Cauliflower Rice	91. Turkey Roll-Ups with Cream Cheese

DAY	BREAKFAST	LUNCH	DINNER	SNACK
Day 42	6. Almond Flour Pancakes	18. Thai Chicken Lettuce Wraps	63. Steak Salad with Avocado	93. Sunflower Seeds with Hard-Boiled Egg
Day 43	9. Low-Carb Breakfast Burrito	14. Zucchini Fritters with Egg	65. Low-Carb Beef Stir-Fry	95. Cottage Cheese with Cucumber Slices
Day 44	13. Low-Carb Granola with Nuts and Seeds	23. Turkey and Veggie Roll-ups	64. Grilled Halibut with Asparagus	99. Low-Carb Lemon Bars
Day 45	7. Smoked Salmon & Cream Cheese Roll	19. Grilled Turkey and Spinach Salad	66. Lemon Herb Chicken Skewers	96. Protein Bars (Homemade)
Day 46	1. Classic Protein Omelette	21. Greek Chicken Salad with Feta	50. Eggplant Lasagna	84. Tropical Mango Smoothie
Day 47	5. Greek Yogurt Protein Parfait	17. Zoodle Salad with Grilled Chicken	41. Grilled Lemon Garlic Salmon	90. Raspberry Chia Pudding
Day 48	14. Zucchini Fritters with Egg	11. Grilled Lemon Garlic Chicken Salad	69. Baked Herb-Crusted Salmon	97. Roasted Pumpkin Seeds
Day 49	2. Low-Carb Breakfast Casserole	24. Mediterranean Chickpea Salad (Low-Carb)	61. Creamy Spinach-Stuffed Chicken Breast	100. Almond Flour Blueberry Muffin
Day 50	10. Chia Seed Pudding with Berries	26. Tuna and Avocado Salad	52. Shrimp Scampi with Zoodles	92. Celery Sticks with Almond Butter
Day 51	6. Almond Flour Pancakes	12. Turkey and Cheese Breakfast Wrap	45. Zoodle Spaghetti with Turkey Meatballs	82. Chocolate Peanut Butter Smoothie
Day 52	3. Avocado and Egg Bowl	13. Low-Carb Granola with Nuts and Seeds	53. Lemon Butter Grilled Chicken	94. Almond Flour Crackers with Guacamole

DAY	BREAKFAST	LUNCH	DINNER	SNACK
Day 53	9. Low-Carb Breakfast Burrito	8. Spinach and Feta Frittata	57. Stir-Fried Tofu with Veggies	85. Blueberry and Kale Smoothie
Day 54	5. Greek Yogurt Protein Parfait	14. Zucchini Fritters with Egg	54. Low-Carb Chicken Alfredo	81. Green Power Smoothie
Day 55	1. Classic Protein Omelette	9. Low-Carb Breakfast Burrito	67. Low-Carb Chicken Enchiladas (No Tortillas)	74. Greek Yogurt with Flaxseeds
Day 56	13. Low-Carb Granola with Nuts and Seeds	25. Grilled Chicken Caesar Salad	60. Low-Carb Beef and Veggie Casserole	72. Veggie Sticks with Hummus
Day 57	2. Low-Carb Breakfast Casserole	16. Caprese Salad with Chicken	64. Grilled Halibut with Asparagus	99. Low-Carb Lemon Bars
Day 58	10. Chia Seed Pudding with Berries	23. Turkey and Veggie Roll-ups	62. Chicken Curry with Cauliflower Rice	76. Cucumber and Tuna Bites
Day 59	4. Egg Muffins with Veggies	18. Thai Chicken Lettuce Wraps	63. Steak Salad with Avocado	78. Spicy Roasted Chickpeas
Day 60	7. Smoked Salmon & Cream Cheese Roll	21. Greek Chicken Salad with Feta	43. Baked Cod with Lemon and Herbs	96. Protein Bars (Homemade)

CONCLUSION
Staying Committed to Your Health

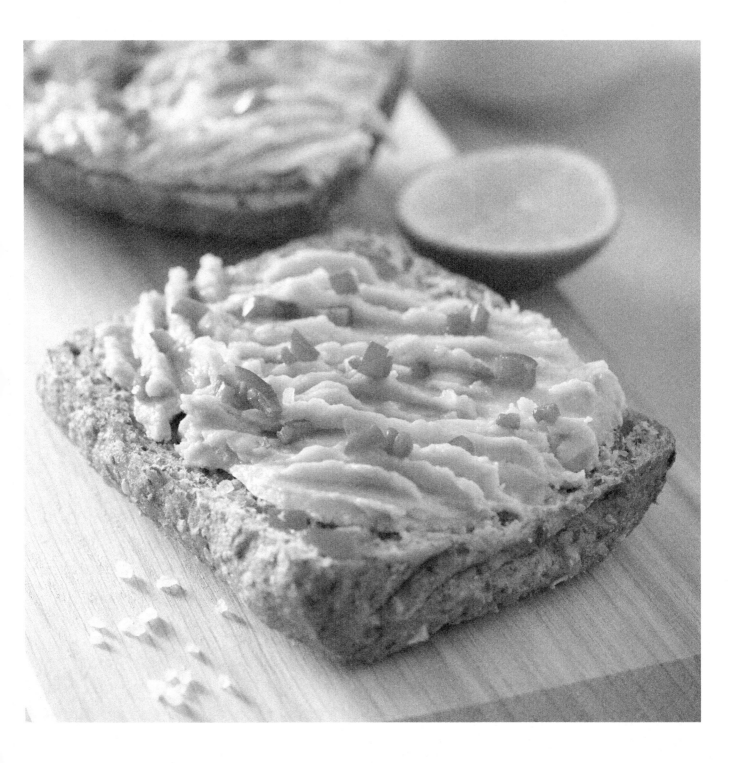

As you reach the end of this 60-day plan, it's important to look back on how far you've come. Committing to a healthier lifestyle, especially one that focuses on balanced nutrition, requires dedication and persistence. The past two months may have brought challenges, but every step you took was a valuable one. Whether you've achieved weight loss, built muscle, or simply found more energy in your day-to-day life, the journey toward better health doesn't stop here. The habits you've started are the foundation for ongoing success.

Now is a perfect time to pause and reflect on what this journey has meant for you personally. Maybe the biggest change is how your clothes fit, or maybe it's the feeling of having more control over your meals and energy levels. The results are not just about physical transformation; they're also about mental shifts. Perhaps you feel more confident, less overwhelmed by meal planning, or more mindful about what you put in your body. These changes are just as important, if not more so, than any number on the scale.

Think back to the beginning of this process and consider how your daily routines have evolved. What new habits have you built? Have you found ways to incorporate meal prep into your weekly schedule? Have you discovered favorite recipes that make healthy eating enjoyable rather than a chore? Reflecting on these questions can help reinforce the positive changes you've made and keep you motivated moving forward.

Of course, it's also important to celebrate the progress you've made. Achievements come in all sizes, and sometimes the small victories—like sticking to your meal plan for an entire week or finding a snack that keeps you satisfied without added sugar—are the ones that matter most. Every healthy decision, no matter how small, is a step toward a better you. By acknowledging your successes, you reinforce the behaviors that led to them, making it easier to stay on track in the future.

Rewarding yourself for these accomplishments is a great way to stay motivated. But instead of turning to food as a reward, consider other ways to celebrate. You might treat yourself to a new kitchen gadget that makes meal prep more fun, plan a relaxing weekend, or even invest in some fitness gear to support your workout routine. Celebrating your progress in ways that align with your goals helps reinforce the new, healthier lifestyle you've built.

Looking ahead, maintaining these healthy habits will be key. While the structured 60-day plan has given you a solid framework, real success lies in your ability to carry these practices forward. To help with this, you'll find several resources that can support your ongoing journey. For instance, the **Quick Low-Carb Snack Guide** offers plenty of easy options to keep hunger at bay without derailing your progress. Having healthy snacks on hand can make all the difference when you're pressed for time or tempted by less nutritious choices.

Additionally, you have access to a **Weekly Meal Planning Template**, which can help you stay organized. Taking the time to plan your meals at the start of each week ensures that you're always prepared, reducing the likelihood of grabbing unhealthy options in a moment of stress or indecision. Meal planning isn't just about discipline—it's about making life easier for yourself in the long run.

If you're cooking for others, the **Family-Friendly Recipe Collection** is designed to help you create meals that everyone will enjoy. This collection ensures you don't need to make separate meals for yourself and your family, making it easier to stick to your plan while satisfying everyone at the table. Integrating these meals into your regular routine can help you maintain your progress without added stress.

As you move forward, remember that perfection isn't the goal—consistency is. There will be days when life gets hectic, and you might miss a workout or grab a quick meal that's not part of the plan. That's okay. What matters is that you don't let these moments derail your overall commitment. The key to long-term success is getting back on track and continuing to make positive choices, even after a slip-up.

You've come a long way in these 60 days, and the habits you've built will serve you well in the months and years to come. Keep experimenting with new recipes, exploring meal prep strategies, and listening to your body's needs. Each day is another opportunity to continue building on the foundation you've created.

Most importantly, be kind to yourself. Progress is not always linear, and it's okay to have ups and downs. The important thing is that you keep moving forward, one healthy choice at a time. You've already proven that you can make significant changes, and now it's about sustaining them.

With the tools and resources you now have at your disposal, you're well-equipped to continue this journey with confidence. Whether your goals are to lose more weight, build more muscle, or simply maintain the progress you've made, you have everything you need to succeed. Here's to your ongoing health, energy, and strength—one meal at a time.

GET YOUR EXCLUSIVE BONUS NOW!

Elevate Your Low-Carb Dieting Experience

With 3 Exclusive BONUS:

1. **Quick Low-Carb Snack Guide**

2. **Weekly Meal Planning Template**

3. **Family-Friendly Recipe Collection**

- THIS BONUS IS 100% FREE -

SCAN THE QR CODE BELOW

Index of Recipes

Printed in Great Britain
by Amazon

56884891R00064